ARTERIAL BLOOD GASES MADE EASY

Iain A M Hennessey MBChB (Hons) BSc (Hons) MRCS

Senior House Officer, Neonatal Intensive Care
Royal United Hospital, Bath, UK

Alan G Japp MBChB (Hons) BSc (Hons) MRCP

Clinical Research Fellow in Cardiology
University of Edinburgh, UK

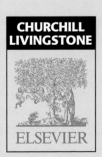

CHURCHILL LIVINGSTONE

ELSEVIER

Edinburgh   London   New York   Oxford   Philadelphia   St Louis   Sydney   Toronto   2007

CHURCHILL
LIVINGSTONE
ELSEVIER

© 2007, Elsevier Limited. All rights reserved.

No part of this publication may be reproduced, stored in a retrieval system, or transmitted in any form or by any means, electronic, mechanical, photocopying, recording or otherwise, without the prior permission of the Publishers. Permissions may be sought directly from Elsevier's Health Sciences Rights Department, 1600 John F. Kennedy Boulevard, Suite 1800, Philadelphia, PA 19103-2899, USA: phone: (+1) 215 239 3804; fax: (+1) 215 239 3805; or, e-mail: *healthpermissions@elsevier.com*. You may also complete your request on-line via the Elsevier homepage (http://www.elsevier.com), by selecting 'Support and contact' and then 'Copyright and Permission'.

First published 2007

ISBN-13: 978-0-443-10414-5 (Main Edition)
ISBN-13: 978-0-443-104138 (International Edition)

British Library Cataloguing in Publication Data
A catalogue record for this book is available from the British Library

Library of Congress Cataloging in Publication Data
A catalog record for this book is available from the Library of Congress

Notice
Neither the publisher nor the authors assume any responsibility for any loss or injury and/or damage to persons or property arising out of or related to any use of the material contained in this book. It is the responsibility of the treating practitioner, relying on independent expertise and knowledge of the patient, to determine the best treatment and method of application for the patient.

The Publisher

Working together to grow
libraries in developing countries

www.elsevier.com | www.bookaid.org | www.sabre.org

ELSEVIER | **BOOK AID** International | **Sabre Foundation**

ELSEVIER | your source for books, journals and multimedia in the health sciences

www.elsevierhealth.com

The publisher's policy is to use **paper manufactured from sustainable forests**

Printed in China

Preface

If you've taken the time to open *Arterial Blood Gases Made Easy*, you must believe that arterial blood gases (ABGs) are important, but not entirely straightforward.

We certainly agree on the first point: ABG analysis now plays an indispensable role in the assessment and management of patients with a huge range of acute medical and surgical problems. Accurate ABG interpretation is undoubtedly a fundamental skill in modern clinical medicine.

On the second point, we hope this book can be of assistance. Throughout, our aims have been to emphasise the key concepts, focus on practical and useful aspects of ABG analysis and avoid extraneous detail. We believe many medical and nursing students, junior doctors and specialist nurses will benefit from a clear, concise guide to performing the technique and interpreting the results.

Iain A M Hennessey
Alan G Japp

Acknowledgements

We are indebted to Dr J K Baillie for his advice, suggestions and constructive criticism and thoroughly recommend a visit to his ABG website, www.altitudephysiology.org. We also wish to thank Dr Jeff Handel for his help and advice, and all others who volunteered ideas, comments or assistance.

Finally we are grateful to Laurence Hunter, Helen Leng and Nancy Arnott for their unfailing support and patience.

Contents

PART 1

THE ABG
EXPLAINED

INTRODUCTION

Arterial blood gas (ABG) analysis refers to the measurement of pH and the *partial pressures* of oxygen (O_2) and carbon dioxide (CO_2) in arterial blood. From these values we can assess the state of *acid–base balance* in blood and how well lungs are performing their job of *gas exchange*.

Already there are questions: what is meant by 'acid–base status'? What is a 'partial pressure'? Why do they matter? It helps to break things down.

Part 1 of this book is designed to answer these questions. We start with a few pages covering the basic essentials of respiratory and acid base physiology: *please do not skip them!* If you understand these core concepts, the rest will follow seamlessly. Part 1 also explains how, when and why to obtain an ABG sample, before concluding with a simple step-by-step guide to interpreting ABG data.

Part 2 then allows you to put all of this into practice with a series of case scenarios involving ABG analysis. You may already have a method for interpreting ABGs but we urge you to try our system (set out in section 1.9) that offers a logical, methodical and consistent way of approaching ABGs. By seeing how this system can identify all of the major patterns of ABG abnormalities, we hope you will gain the necessary confidence to apply it in clinical practice.

PULMONARY GAS EXCHANGE: THE BASICS

Our cells use oxygen (O_2) to generate energy and produce carbon dioxide (CO_2) as waste. Blood supplies cells with the O_2 they need and clears the unwanted CO_2. This process depends on the ability of our lungs to enrich blood with O_2 and rid it of CO_2.

Pulmonary gas exchange refers to the transfer of O_2 from the atmosphere to the bloodstream (oxygenation) and CO_2 from the bloodstream to the atmosphere (CO_2 elimination).

The exchange takes place between tiny air sacs called *alveoli* and blood vessels called *capillaries*. Because they each have extremely thin walls and come into very close contact (the alveolar–capillary membrane), CO_2 and O_2 are able to move (*diffuse*) between them (Figure 1).

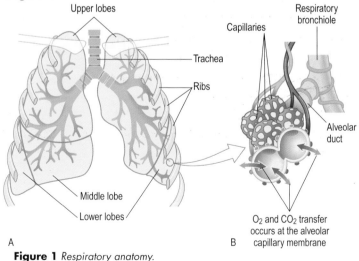

Figure 1 *Respiratory anatomy.*

PULMONARY GAS EXCHANGE: PARTIAL PRESSURES

ABGs help us to assess the effectiveness of gas exchange by providing measurements of the *partial pressures* of O_2 and CO_2 in arterial blood – the Pa_{O_2} and Pa_{CO_2}.

Partial pressure describes the contribution of one individual gas within a gas mixture (such as air) to the total pressure. When a gas dissolves in liquid (e.g. blood), the amount dissolved depends on the partial pressure.

Note

Po_2 = **partial pressure of O_2**
Pa_{O_2} = **partial pressure of O_2** *in arterial blood*

Gases move from areas of higher partial pressure to lower partial pressure. At the alveolar–capillary membrane, air in alveoli has a higher Po_2 and lower Pco_2 than capillary blood. Thus, O_2 molecules move from alveoli to blood and CO_2 molecules move from blood to alveoli until the partial pressures are equal.

A note on ... gas pressures

At sea level, atmospheric pressure (total pressure of gases in the atmosphere) = 101 kPa or 760 mmHg

O_2 comprises 21% of air, so the partial pressure of O_2 in air
= 21% of atmospheric pressure
= 21 kPa or 160 mmHg

CO_2 makes up just a tiny fraction of air, so the partial pressure of CO_2 in inspired air is negligible

---

CARBON DIOXIDE ELIMINATION

Diffusion of CO_2 from the bloodstream to alveoli is so efficient that CO_2 elimination is actually limited by how quickly we can "blow-off" the CO_2 in our alveoli. Thus, the $PaCO_2$ (which reflects the overall amount of CO_2 in arterial blood) is determined by *alveolar ventilation* – the total volume of air transported between alveoli and the outside world every minute.

Ventilation is regulated by an area in the brainstem called the respiratory centre. This area contains specialised receptors that sense the $PaCO_2$ and connect with the muscles involved in breathing. If it is abnormal, the respiratory centre adjusts the rate and depth of breathing accordingly (Figure 2).

Normally, lungs can maintain a normal $PaCO_2$, even in conditions where CO_2 production is unusually high (e.g. sepsis). Consequently an increased $PaCO_2$ (hypercapnia) always implies reduced alveolar ventilation.

Key point

$PaCO_2$ is controlled by ventilation and the level of ventilation is adjusted to maintain $PaCO_2$ within tight limits.

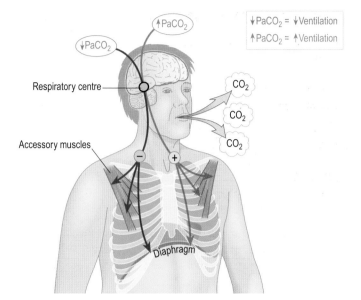

Figure 2 *Control of ventilation.*

A note on ... hypoxic drive

In patients with chronically high $PaCO_2$ levels (chronic hypercapnia), the specialised receptors that detect CO_2 levels can become desensitised. The body then relies on receptors that detect the Pao_2 to gauge the adequacy of ventilation and low Pao_2 becomes the principal ventilatory stimulus. This is referred to as *hypoxic drive*.

In patients who rely on hypoxic drive, overzealous correction of hypoxaemia, with supplemental O_2, may depress ventilation, leading to a catastrophic rise in $PaCO_2$. Patients with chronic hypercapnia must therefore be given supplemental O_2 in a controlled fashion with careful ABG monitoring. The same does not apply to patients with acute hypercapnia.

HAEMOGLOBIN OXYGEN SATURATION (SO_2)

Oxygenation is more complicated than CO_2 elimination. The first thing to realise is that the P_{O_2} does not actually tell us how much O_2 is in blood. It only measures free, unbound O_2 molecules – a tiny proportion of the total.

In fact, almost all O_2 molecules in blood are bound to a protein called *haemoglobin* Hb (Figure 3). Because of this, the amount of O_2 in blood depends on two factors:

1. **Hb concentration:** this determines how much O_2 blood has *the capacity to carry.*

2. **Saturation of Hb with O2 (So_2):** this is the percentage of available binding sites on Hb that contain an O2 molecule – **i.e.** *how much of the carrying capacity is being used* (Figure 4).

Note

So_2 = O_2 saturation in (any) blood
Sao_2 = O_2 saturation in *arterial blood*

A note on ... pulse oximetry

Sao_2 can be measured using a probe (pulse oximeter) applied to the finger or earlobe. In most cases it provides adequate information to gauge oxygenation, but it is less accurate with saturations below 75% and unreliable when peripheral perfusion is poor. Oximetry does not provide information on $Paco_2$ so should not be used as a substitute for ABG analysis in ventilatory impairment.

Key point

Po_2 is not a measure of the amount of O_2 in blood – ultimately the Sao_2 and Hb concentration determine the O_2 content of arterial blood.

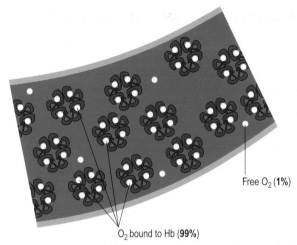

Figure 3 *Relative proportions of free O_2 molecules and O_2 molecules bound to haemoglobin in blood.*

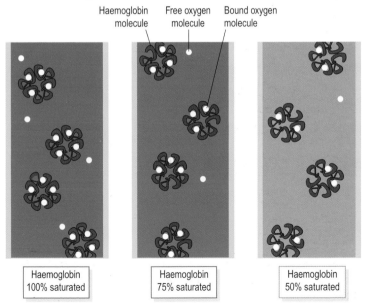

Figure 4 *Haemoglobin oxygen saturation.*

OXYHAEMOGLOBIN DISSOCIATION CURVE

We now know that the amount of O_2 in blood depends on the Hb concentration and the S_{O_2}. So what is the significance of the P_{O_2}?

P_{O_2} can be thought of as the driving force for O_2 molecules to bind to Hb: as such it regulates the S_{O_2}. The oxyhaemoglobin dissociation curve (Figure 5) shows the S_{O_2} that will result from any given P_{O_2}.

In general, the higher the P_{O_2}, the higher the S_{O_2}, but *the curve is not linear*. The green line is known as the 'flat part of the curve': changes in P_{O_2} over this range have relatively little effect on the S_{O_2}. In contrast, the red line is known as the 'steep part of the curve': even small changes in P_{O_2} over this range may have a major impact on S_{O_2}.

Note that, with a 'normal' Pa_{O_2} of around 13 kPa (100 mmHg), Hb is, more or less, *maximally saturated* ($Sa_{O_2} > 95\%$). This means blood has used up its O_2-carrying capacity and any further rise in Pa_{O_2} will *not* significantly increase arterial O_2 content.

Key point

P_{O_2} is not the amount of O_2 in blood but is the driving force for saturating Hb with O_2.

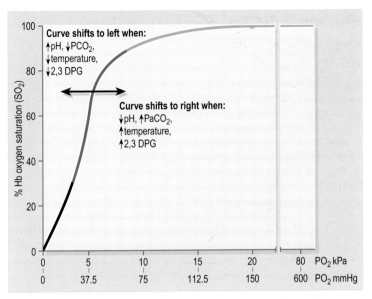

Figure 5 *Oxyhaemoglobin dissociation curve. The curve defines the relationship between Po_2 and the percentage saturation of haemoglobin with oxygen (So_2). Note the sigmoid shape: it is relatively flat when Po_2 is > 80 mmHg (10.6 kPa) but steep when Po_2 falls below 60 mmHg (8 kPa).*

Key point

When Hb approaches maximal O_2 saturation, further increases in Po_2 do not significantly increase blood O_2 content.

ALVEOLAR VENTILATION AND PaO_2

We have now seen how Pa_{O_2} regulates the Sa_{O_2}. But what determines Pa_{O_2}?

There are three major factors that dictate the Pa_{O_2}:

1. **Alveolar ventilation**

2. **Matching of ventilation with perfusion (V/Q)**

3. **Concentration of O_2 in inspired air (Fi_{O_2})**

Alveolar ventilation

O_2 moves rapidly from alveoli to the bloodstream – so *the higher the alveolar P_{O_2}, the higher the Pa_{O_2}.*

Unlike air in the atmosphere, alveolar air contains significant amounts of CO_2 (Figure 6). More CO_2 means a lower P_{O_2} (remember the partial pressure of a gas reflects its share of the total volume).

An increase in alveolar ventilation allows more CO_2 to be 'blown off', resulting in a higher alveolar P_{O_2}. If, on the other hand, ventilation declines, CO_2 accumulates at the expense of O_2 and alveolar P_{O_2} falls.

Whereas hyperventiation can increase alveolar P_{O_2} only slightly (bringing it closer to the P_{O_2} of inspired air), there is no limit to how far alveolar P_{O_2} (and hence Pa_{O_2}) can fall with inadequate ventilation.

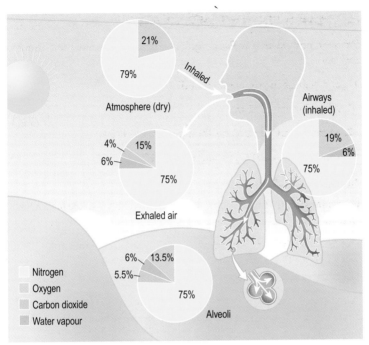

Figure 6 *Composition of inhaled and exhaled gases at various stages of respiration.*

Key point

Both oxygenation and CO_2 elimination depend on alveolar ventilation: impaired ventilation causes Pa_{O_2} to fall and Pa_{CO_2} to rise.

Ventilation/perfusion mismatch and shunting

Not all blood flowing through the lung meets well-ventilated alveoli and not all ventilated alveoli are perfused with blood – especially in the presence of lung disease. This problem is known as ventilation/perfusion (V/Q) mismatch.

Imagine if alveoli in one area of lung are poorly ventilated (e.g. due to collapse or consolidation). Blood passing these alveoli returns to the arterial circulation with less O_2 and more CO_2 than normal. This is known as *shunting*[1].

Now, by *hyperventilating*, we can shift more air in and out of our remaining 'good alveoli'. This allows them to blow-off extra CO_2 so that the blood passing them can offload more CO_2. The lower CO_2 in non-shunted blood compensates for the higher CO_2 in shunted blood, maintaining the $PaCO_2$.

The same does NOT apply to oxygenation. Blood passing 'good alveoli' is not able to carry more O_2 because its haemoglobin is already maximally saturated with O_2 (remember: flat part of curve, page 11). The non-shunted blood therefore cannot compensate for the low O_2 levels in shunted blood and the PaO_2 falls.

Key point

V/Q mismatch allows poorly oxygenated blood to re-enter the arterial circulation, thus lowering Pa_{O_2} and Sa_{O_2}.

Provided overall alveolar ventilation is maintained, V/Q mismatch does not lead to an increase in Pa_{CO_2}.

---

[1]The term also applies to blood that bypasses alveoli altogether (anatomical shunting)

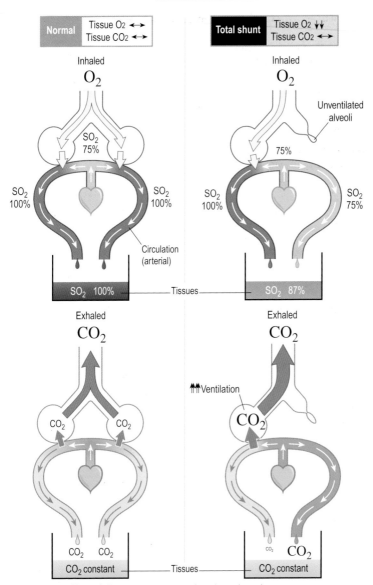

Figure 7 Effect of shunt on oxygen and carbon dioxide.

Fio_2 and oxygenation

The fraction of inspired oxygen (FiO_2) refers to the percentage of O_2 in the air we breathe in. The FiO_2 in room air is 21%, but can be increased with supplemental O_2.

A low PaO_2 may result from either V/Q mismatch or inadequate ventilation and, in both cases, increasing the FiO_2 will improve the PaO_2. The exact FiO_2 requirement varies depending on how severely oxygenation is impaired and will help to determine the choice of delivery device (Figure 8). When the cause is inadequate ventilation it must be remembered that increasing FiO_2 will not reverse the rise in $PaCO_2$.

Supplemental O_2 makes ABG analysis more complex as it can be difficult to judge whether the PaO_2 is appropriately high for the Fio_2 and, hence, whether oxygenation is impaired. A useful rule of thumb is that the difference between FiO_2 and PaO_2 (in kPa) should not normally be greater than 10. However there is often a degree of uncertainty as to the precise FiO_2 and, if subtle impairment is suspected, the ABG should be repeated on room air.

Oxygen delivery devices

Nasal prongs: FiO_2 < 40%. Comfortable and convenient. FiO_2 non-specific: depends on flow rate (1–6 L/min) and ventilation

Standard face mask: FiO_2 30–50% at flow rates 6–10 L/min but imprecise. May cause CO_2 retention at flows < 5 L/min ('rebreathing'), so not useful for providing lower FiO_2.

Fixed performance (high-flow) face mask: FiO_2 24–60%. Delivers fixed, predictable FiO_2. Ideal for providing controlled, accurate O_2 therapy at low concentrations.

Face mask with reservoir: FiO_2 60–80%. Can achieve even higher FiO_2 with tight-fitting mask. Useful for short-term use in respiratory emergencies.

Endotracheal intubation: FiO_2 21–100%. Used in severely unwell patients with very high O_2 requirements, especially with ventilatory failure. Patient is sedated and mechanically ventilated.

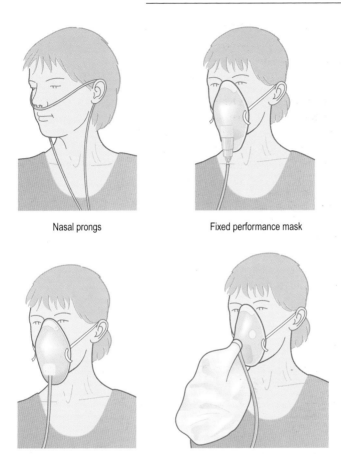

Nasal prongs

Fixed performance mask

Variable performance mask

Mask with reservoir

Figure 8 *Oxygen delivery devices.*

DISORDERS OF GAS EXCHANGE

HYPOXIA, HYPOXAEMIA AND IMPAIRED OXYGENATION

The above terms are often used interchangeably but mean different things.

Hypoxia refers to *any state in which tissues receive an inadequate supply of O_2 to support normal aerobic metabolism*[1] (Figure 9). It may result from either hypoxaemia (see below) or impaired blood supply to tissues (ischaemia). It is often associated with lactic acidosis as cells resort to anaerobic metabolism.

Hypoxaemia refers to *any state in which the O_2 content of arterial blood is reduced*. It may result from impaired oxygenation (see below), low haemoglobin (anaemia) or reduced affinity of haemoglobin for O_2 (e.g. carbon monoxide).

Impaired oxygenation refers to *hypoxaemia resulting from reduced transfer of O_2 from lungs to the bloodstream*. It is identified by a low Pa_{O_2} (< 10.7 kPa; < 80 mmHg).

It is important to note the distinction between *impaired* oxygenation (which results in hypoxaemia) and *inadequate* oxygenation (which results in hypoxia). Consider a patient with a Pa_{O_2} of 8.5 kPa. He has impaired oxygenation, suggesting the presence of important lung disease. Nevertheless, his Pa_{O_2} would usually result in an Sa_{O_2} > 90% and, *provided the haemoglobin and cardiac output are normal*, adequate O_2 delivery to tissues.

---

[1]It is often advisable to use the term 'tissue hypoxia' to avoid any confusion.

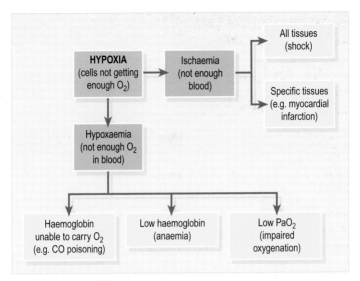

Figure 9 *Causes of hypoxia.*

TYPE 1 RESPIRATORY IMPAIRMENT

Type 1 respiratory impairment[1] is defined as low Pa_{O_2} with normal or low Pa_{CO_2}. This implies defective oxygenation despite adequate ventilation. V/Q mismatch is usually responsible and may result from a number of causes (Box 1.3.1). The Pa_{CO_2} is often low due to compensatory hyperventilation.

If the ABG is drawn from a patient on supplemental O_2, the Pa_{O_2} may not be below the normal range, but will be inappropriately low for the Fi_{O_2}.

The severity of type 1 respiratory impairment is judged according to the scale of the resulting hypoxaemia and, ultimately, the presence of hypoxia (Table 1.3.1). Here it is important to remember the O_2 dissociation curve. Reductions in Pa_{O_2} as far as 8 kPa have a relatively minor effect on Sa_{O_2} and are well tolerated. Beyond this threshold, we reach the 'steep part' of the curve and further reductions in Pa_{O_2} will lead to much greater falls in Sa_{O_2}, significantly lowering the O_2 content of arterial blood.

Initial treatment of type 1 respiratory impairment is aimed at achieving an adequate Pa_{O_2} and Sa_{O_2} with supplemental O_2 while attempting to correct the underlying cause. In many cases pulse oximetry can be used as an alternative to repeated ABG sampling to monitor progress.

---

[1]We use the term 'impairment' rather than 'failure' here as the diagnosis of respiratory failure requires a $Pa_{O_2} < 8$ kPa (< 60 mmHg).

Box 1.3.1   Common causes of type 1 respiratory impairment*

Pneumonia	Acute asthma
Pulmonary embolism	Acute respiratory distress syndrome
Pneumothorax	Fibrosing alveolitis
Pulmonary oedema	Chronic obstructive pulmonary disease

*The usual mechanism is V/Q mismatch; however, some conditions (e.g. alveolitis) impair diffusion of gases across the alveolar capillary membrane.

Table 1.3.1   Assessing severity of type 1 respiratory impairment

	Mild	Moderate	Severe
Pao_2 (kPa)	8–10.6	5.3–7.9	< 5.3
Pao_2 (mmHg)	60–79	40–59	< 40
Sao_2 (%)	90–94	75–89	< 75

Other markers of severe impairment

- High Fio_2 requirements to maintain adequate Pao_2
- Lactic acidosis (indicating tissue hypoxia)
- Organ dysfunction (drowsiness, confusion, renal failure, haemodynamic collapse, coma)

TYPE 2 RESPIRATORY IMPAIRMENT

Type 2 respiratory impairment is defined by a high Pa_{CO_2} (hypercapnia) and is due to inadequate alveolar ventilation. Since oxygenation also depends on ventilation, the Pa_{O_2} is usually low, but may be normal if the patient is on supplemental O_2. It is important to note that any cause of type 1 impairment may lead to type 2 impairment if exhaustion supervenes.

Acute rises in Pa_{CO_2} lead to dangerous accumulation of acid in the blood (see section 1.4) and must be reversed. Chronic hypercapnia is accompanied by a rise in bicarbonate (HCO_3), which preserves acid–base balance. However, patients with chronic type 2 impairment who experience a further sharp decline in ventilation will also have a rapid rise in Pa_{CO_2} (acute on chronic), leading to acid accumulation and low blood pH (Table 1.3.2).

Supplemental O_2 improves hypoxaemia but not hypercapnia, so treatment of type 2 respiratory impairment should also include measures to improve ventilation (e.g. reversal of sedation, relief of airways obstruction, assisted ventilation). The overzealous administration of supplemental O_2 to some patients with *chronic* type 2 impairment may further depress ventilation by abolishing hypoxic drive (p. 7).

Pulse oximetry provides no information on Pa_{CO_2} so is not a suitable substitute for ABG monitoring in type 2 respiratory impairment.

Table 1.3.2 The ABG in different patterns of type 2 impairment

	Pa_{CO_2}	HCO_3	pH
Acute	↑	→	↓
Chronic	↑	↑	→
Acute on chronic	↑	↑	↓

Box 1.3.2 Common causes of type 2 respiratory impairment

Chronic obstructive pulmonary disease*	Opiate/benzodiazepine toxicity
Exhaustion	Inhaled foreign body
Flail chest injury	Neuromuscular disorders
Kyphoscoliosis	Obstructive sleep apnoea

*May lead to either type 1 or type 2 respiratory impairment

Box 1.3.3 Clinical signs of hypercapnia

Confusion	Drowsiness
Flapping tremor	Bounding pulse
Warm extremities	Headache

HYPERVENTILATION

Hyperventilation leads to a low $Pa\text{CO}_2$ (hypocapnia) and a corresponding rise in blood pH (see section 1.4). In chronic cases it is accompanied by a rise in HCO_3, which corrects blood pH. An increase in the rate and depth of breathing is usually apparent. A large drop in $Pa\text{CO}_2$ may lead to tingling around the mouth and extremities, light-headedness and even syncope.

Psychogenic hyperventilation often presents in a dramatic fashion, with patients complaining of severe breathlessness and an inability to take in enough air. It may be difficult to distinguish from respiratory disease. The ABG shows a low $Pa\text{CO}_2$ with a normal $Pa\text{O}_2$.

Hyperventilation also occurs as a compensatory response to metabolic acidosis (secondary hyperventilation), as described in section 1.4. Other causes are shown in Table 1.3.3.

Table 1.3.3	Common causes of hyperventilation	
Primary	Anxiety (psychogenic)	Pain or distress
	Hypoxaemia	Fever
	Salicylate toxicity	Central nervous system disorders
	Hepatic cirrhosis	
Secondary	Metabolic acidosis (of any aetiology)	

SUMMARY OF GAS EXCHANGE ABNORMALITIES

The four main patterns of ABG abnormality in disorders of gas exchange are summarised in Table 1.3.4.

Table 1.3.4			
	Pao_2	$Paco_2$	HCO_3
Respiratory impairment			
Type 1	↓	↓/→	→
Acute type 2	↓/→	↑	→
Chronic type 2*	↓/→	↑	↑
Hyperventilation	→	↓	→/↓

*Acute on chronic distinguished from chronic by presence of ↑ H^+.

A note on ... the A–a gradient

The A–a gradient is the difference between the alveolar Po_2 (averaged across all alveoli) and the Po_2 in arterial blood. It tells us whether the Pao_2 is appropriate for the level of alveolar ventilation and is therefore a measure of the degree of V/Q mismatch.

In practice its main uses lie in detecting subtle increases in V/Q mismatch where the Pao_2 is still within the normal range (e.g. pulmonary embolism) and identifying the presence of V/Q mismatch in patients with type 2 respiratory impairment (this distinguishes pure type 2 respiratory impairment from mixed type 1 and type 2 impairment).

Calculation of the A–a gradient is not required for the scenarios in Part 2 of the book but, for those interested, a guide can be found in Appendix 1.

ACID–BASE BALANCE: THE BASICS

The terms acidity and alkalinity simply refer to the concentration of free hydrogen ions (H^+) in a solution. H^+ concentration can be expressed directly in nanomoles per litre (nmol/L) or as pH (see over).

Solutions with high H^+ (low pH) are acidic and those with low H^+ (high pH) are alkaline. The point at which a substance changes from alkali to acid is the neutral point (pH = 7, H^+ = 100 nmol/L).

An acid is a substance that *releases* H^+ when it is dissolved in solution. Acids therefore increase the H^+ concentration of the solution (lower the pH). A base is a substance that *accepts* H^+ when dissolved in solution. Bases therefore lower the H^+ concentration of a solution (raise the pH). A buffer is a substance that can either accept or release H^+ depending on the surrounding H^+ concentration. Buffers therefore resist big changes in H^+ concentration.

Human blood normally has a pH of 7.35–7.45 (H^+ = 35–45 nmol/L) so is slightly alkaline. If blood pH is below the normal range (< 7.35), there is an acidaemia. If it is above the normal range (> 7.45), there is an alkalaemia.

An acidosis is any process that lowers blood pH whereas an alkalosis is any process that raises blood pH.

What is pH?

The pH (power of hydrogen) scale is a simplified way of expressing large changes in H^+ concentration, though if you've not come across it before you might think it was designed just to confuse you!

It is a *negative logarithmic* scale (Figure 10). The 'negative' means that pH values get lower as the H^+ concentration increases (so a pH of 7.1 is more acidic than 7.2). The 'logarithmic' means that a shift in pH by one number represents a 10-fold change in H^+ concentration (so 7 is *10 times* more acidic than 8).

Why is acid–base balance important?

For cellular processes to occur efficiently, the H^+ concentration must be kept within tight limits. Failure to maintain pH balance leads to inefficient cellular reactions and ultimately death (Figure 10).

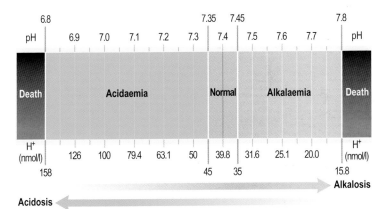

Figure 10 *pH/H$^+$ scale.*

MAINTAINING ACID–BASE BALANCE

What generates H⁺ ions in our bodies?

The breakdown of fats and sugars for energy generates CO_2 which, when dissolved in blood, forms carbonic acid (see Box on page 29).

Metabolism of protein produces hydrochloric, sulphuric and other so-called 'metabolic acids'.

H^+ ions must, therefore, be removed to maintain normal blood pH.

What removes H⁺ ions from our bodies?

Respiratory mechanisms

Our lungs are responsible for removing CO_2. Pa_{CO_2}, the partial pressure of carbon dioxide in our blood, is determined by alveolar ventilation. If CO_2 production is altered, we adjust our breathing to exhale more or less CO_2, as necessary, to maintain Pa_{CO_2} within normal limits. The bulk of the acid produced by our bodies is in the form of CO_2, so it is our lungs that excrete the vast majority of the acid load.

Renal (metabolic) mechanisms

The kidneys are responsible for excreting metabolic acids. They secrete H^+ ions into urine and reabsorb HCO_3 from urine. HCO_3 is a base (and therefore accepts H^+ ions), so it reduces the concentration of H^+ ions in blood. The kidneys can adjust urinary H^+ and HCO_3 excretion in response to changes in metabolic acid production.

MAINTAINING ACID–BASE BALANCE

The renal and respiratory systems operate jointly to maintain blood pH within normal limits. If one system is overwhelmed, leading to a change in blood pH, the other usually adjusts, automatically, to limit the disturbance (e.g. if kidneys fail to excrete metabolic acids, ventilation is increased to exhale more CO_2). This is known as *compensation*.

Importantly, compensatory changes in respiration happen over minutes to hours, whereas metabolic responses take days to develop.

Just one equation...

This one equation is crucial to understanding acid–base balance:

$$H_2O + CO_2 \leftrightarrow H_2CO_3 \leftrightarrow H^+ + HCO_3^-$$

Firstly it shows that CO_2, when dissolved in blood, becomes an acid.

The more CO_2 added to blood, the more H_2CO_3 (carbonic acid) is produced, which dissociates to release free H^+ ions.

Secondly, it predicts that blood pH depends not on the absolute amounts of CO_2 or HCO_3 present but on *the ratio of CO_2 to HCO_3*. Thus, a change in CO_2 will not lead to a change in pH if it is balanced by a change in HCO_3 that preserves the ratio (and vice versa). Since CO_2 is controlled by respiration and HCO_3 by renal excretion, this explains how compensation can prevent changes in blood pH.

DISTURBANCES OF ACID–BASE BALANCE

An acidosis is any process that acts to lower blood pH. If it is due to a rise in Pa_{CO_2}, it is called a *respiratory acidosis*; if it is due to any other cause, then HCO_3 is reduced and it is called a *metabolic acidosis*.

An alkalosis is any process that acts to increase blood pH. If it is due to a fall in Pa_{CO_2}, it is called a *respiratory alkalosis*; if it is due to any other cause, then HCO_3 is raised and it is called a *metabolic alkalosis*.

Pa_{CO_2} raised	=	Respiratory acidosis
Pa_{CO_2} low	=	Respiratory alkalosis
HCO_3 raised	=	Metabolic alkalosis
HCO_3 low	=	Metabolic acidosis

Acid–base disturbances can be considered as a set of scales.

Normal acid–base balance

When acid–base balance is entirely normal, with no alkalotic or acidotic pressures, it is like having a set of scales with no weights on it (Figure 11).

Uncompensated acid–base disturbance

When an acidosis or alkalosis develops, the scales become unbalanced, leading to acidaemia or alkalaemia respectively.
In Figure 12 there is a primary respiratory acidosis with no opposing metabolic process.

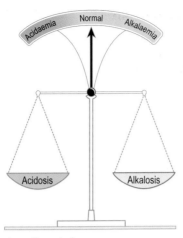

Figure 11 *Normal acid-base balance.*

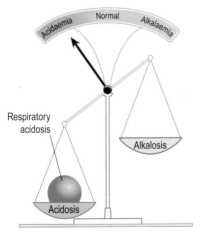

Figure 12 *Uncompensated respiratory acidosis.*

COMPENSATED ACID–BASE DISTURBANCE

As described earlier, a respiratory or metabolic disturbance is often *compensated* for by adjustment of the other system to offset the primary disturbance.

Figures 13 and 14 represent two scenarios in which the lungs have responded to a primary metabolic acidosis by increasing alveolar ventilation to eliminate more CO_2 (compensatory respiratory alkalosis). In Figure 13 an acidaemia persists despite compensation (partial compensation); in Figure 14, blood pH has returned to the normal range (full compensation).

When faced with such an ABG, how can we tell which is the primary disturbance and which is the compensatory process?

The first rule to remember is that *overcompensation does not occur*. The midpoint of the acid–base scales lies at a pH of 7.4 (H^+ 40). If the scales tip toward acidaemia (pH < 7.4), this suggests a primary acidotic process; if they tip toward alkalaemia (pH > 7.4), a primary alkalotic process is likely.

The second rule is that *the patient is more important than the ABG*. When considering an ABG, one must always take account of the clinical context. For example, if the patient in Figure 14 were diabetic, with high levels of ketones in the urine, it would be obvious that the metabolic acidosis was a primary process (diabetic ketoacidosis).

A note on ... predicting compensatory responses

It is not always easy to distinguish two primary opposing processes from a compensated disturbance. A more precise method than that described above involves calculating the expected compensatory response for any given primary disturbance. However these calculations are usually unnecessary and are *not* required for the case scenarios in Part 2.

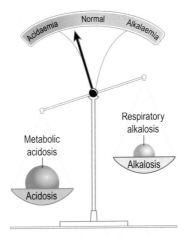

Figure 13 *Partially compensated metabolic acidosis.*

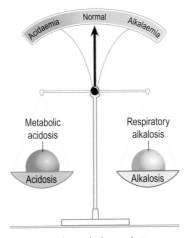

Figure 14 *Fully compensated metabolic acidosis.*

MIXED ACID–BASE DISTURBANCE

When a primary respiratory disturbance and primary metabolic disturbance occur simultaneously there is said to be a *mixed* acid–base disturbance.

If these two processes oppose each other, the pattern will be similar to a compensated acid–base disturbance (Figure 14) and the resulting pH derangement will be minimised. A good example is salicylate poisoning, where primary hyperventilation (respiratory alkalosis) and metabolic acidosis (salicylate is acidic) occur independently.

On the other hand, if the two processes cause pH to move in the same direction (metabolic acidosis and respiratory acidosis *or* metabolic alkalosis and respiratory alkalosis), a profound acidaemia or alkalaemia may result (Figure 15).

The nomogram

An alternative way to analyse ABGs is to use the acid–base nomogram (Figure 16). By plotting the $Pa\text{co}_2$ and H^+/pH values on the ABG nomogram, most ABGs can be analysed. If the plotted point lies outside the designated areas, this implies a mixed disturbance.

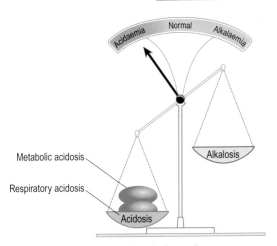

Figure 15 *Mixed respiratory and metabolic acidosis.*

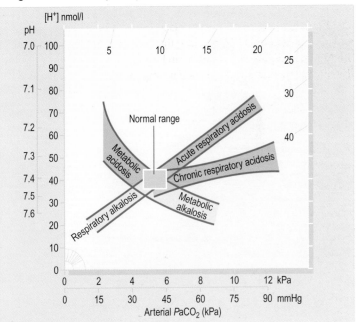

Figure 16 *The nomogram.*

DISORDERS OF ACID–BASE BALANCE

METABOLIC ACIDOSIS

A metabolic acidosis is any process, *other than a rise in* Pa_{CO_2}, that acts to lower blood pH. It may occur through accumulation of metabolic acids (excess ingestion, increased production or reduced renal excretion) or through excessive loss of base (HCO_3). Calculating the anion gap (see over) may help to establish the cause of a metabolic acidosis.

Metabolic acidosis is recognised on an ABG by low HCO_3 (and negative base excess (BE)). There is normally a compensatory increase in alveolar ventilation to lower Pa_{CO_2}. If respiratory compensation is overwhelmed, an acidaemia will result. Severity must be judged according to both the underlying process and the resulting acidaemia. An $HCO_3 < 15$ mmol/L (or BE < 10) indicates a severe acidotic process whereas a pH < 7.25 ($H^+ > 55$) constitutes serious acidaemia.

The dominant symptom in metabolic acidosis is often hyperventilation (Kussmaul's respiration) owing to the respiratory compensation. Other signs are fairly non-specific or related to the underlying cause. Profound acidaemia (pH < 7.15; $H^+ > 70$) may lead to circulatory shock, organ dysfunction, and, ultimately death.

Specific causes of metabolic acidosis are discussed in greater detail in the relevant cases in Part 2.

The anion gap

In blood, positively charged ions (cations) must be balanced by negatively charged ions (anions) to maintain *electroneutrality*. But when the main cations ($Na^+ + K^+$) are compared with the main anions ($Cl^- + HCO_3^-$), there appears to be a shortage of anions or an anion gap.

Anion gap = (Na + K) – (Cl + HCO₃) [Normal = 10 – 18 mmol/L]

The gap is made up of unmeasured anions such as phosphate and sulphate and negatively charged proteins (these are difficult to measure).

A raised anion gap (>18 mmol/L) therefore indicates the presence of increased unmeasured anions, e.g. lactate, salicylate.

A note on ... lactic acidosis

This common cause of metabolic acidosis occurs when tissues receive an inadequate supply of O_2 due to either hypoxaemia or impaired perfusion. Normal aerobic metabolism (which relies on O_2) is then replaced by anaerobic metabolism (which generates lactic acid). Lactic acidosis is therefore a marker of tissue hypoxia and a useful indicator of severity in a variety of conditions, including severe hypoxaemia or shock from any cause.

METABOLIC ALKALOSIS

A metabolic alkalosis is any process, *other than a fall in Pa_{CO_2}*, that acts to increase blood pH and is characterised by a *rise in plasma HCO_3*. Respiratory compensation ($\uparrow Pa_{CO_2}$) occurs to limit the resulting alkalaemia but is limited by the need to avoid hypoxaemia.

Loss of H^+ ions may initiate the process but the kidneys have huge scope to correct threatened alkalosis by increasing HCO_3 excretion. Factors that impair this response are therefore also necessary. The usual suspects are depletion of chloride (Cl^-), potassium (K^+) and sodium (Na^+) ions – in most cases due to either sustained vomiting (Figure 17) or diuretic drugs.

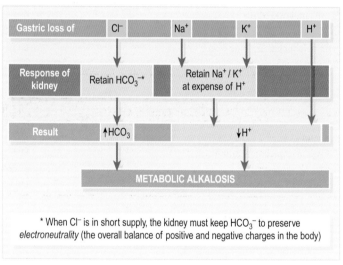

* When Cl^- is in short supply, the kidney must keep HCO_3^- to preserve *electroneutrality* (the overall balance of positive and negative charges in the body)

Figure 17 *Effect of vomiting on acid–base balance.*

SUMMARY OF METABOLIC ACID–BASE DISORDERS

Box 1.5.1 Metabolic acidosis (low HCO₃)

With raised anion gap

Lactic acidosis (e.g. hypoxaemia, shock, sepsis, infarction)
Ketoacidosis (diabetes, starvation, alcohol excess)
Renal failure
Poisoning (aspirin, methanol, ethylene glycol)

With normal anion gap

Renal tubular acidosis
Diarrhoea
Ammonium chloride ingestion
Adrenal insufficiency

Box 1.5.2 Metabolic alkalosis (high HCO₃)

Vomiting
Potassium depletion (e.g. diuretics)
Cushing's syndrome
Conn's syndrome (primary hyperaldosteronism)

RESPIRATORY ACIDOSIS

A respiratory acidosis is, simply, *an increase in* Pa_{CO_2}. Since CO_2 dissolves in blood to form carbonic acid, this has the effect of lowering pH ($\uparrow H^+$ ions).

Normally, lungs are able to increase ventilation to maintain a normal Pa_{CO_2} – even in conditions of increased CO_2 production (e.g. sepsis). Thus, respiratory acidosis always implies a degree of reduced alveolar ventilation. This may occur from any cause of type 2 respiratory impairment (see section 1.3) or to counteract a metabolic alkalosis.

RESPIRATORY ALKALOSIS

A respiratory alkalosis is *a decrease in* Pa_{CO_2} and is caused by alveolar hyperventilation. Primary causes include, pain, anxiety (hyperventilation syndrome), fever, breathlessness and hypoxaemia. It may also occur to counteract a metabolic acidosis.

Acute versus chronic respiratory acidosis

Since metabolic compensatory responses take days to develop, acute respiratory acidosis is almost always *uncompensated*, leading rapidly to profound and dangerous acidaemia. Indeed, an opposing metabolic alkalosis suggests that a respiratory acidosis must have been present for some time. In other words, the presence of metabolic compensation distinguishes chronic from acute type 2 ventilatory failure (see section 1.3).

MIXED RESPIRATORY AND METABOLIC ACIDOSIS

This is the most dangerous pattern of acid–base abnormality. It leads to profound acidaemia as there are two simultaneous acidotic processes with no compensation. In clinical practice it is often due to severe ventilatory failure, in which the rising Pa_{CO_2} (respiratory acidosis) is accompanied by a low Pa_{O_2}, resulting in tissue hypoxia and consequent lactic acidosis.

ABG SAMPLING TECHNIQUE

Before you can interpret an ABG you must, of course, obtain a sample of arterial blood. The following steps should be used as a guide but the best way to learn is at the bedside with experienced supervision.

BEFORE SAMPLING

- Confirm the need for the ABG and identify any contraindications (Box 1.6.1).

- Always record details of O_2 therapy and respiratory support (e.g. ventilator settings).

- Unless results are required urgently, allow at least 20 minutes after any change in O_2 therapy before sampling (to achieve a steady state).

- Explain to the patient why you are doing the test, what it involves and the possible complications (bleeding, bruising, arterial thrombosis, infection and pain); then obtain consent to proceed.

- Prepare the necessary equipment (heparinised syringe with cap, 20–22G needle, sharps disposal container, gauze) and don universal precautions.

- Identify a suitable site for sampling by palpating the radial, brachial or femoral artery (Figure 18). Routine sampling should, initially, be attempted from the radial artery of the non-dominant arm.

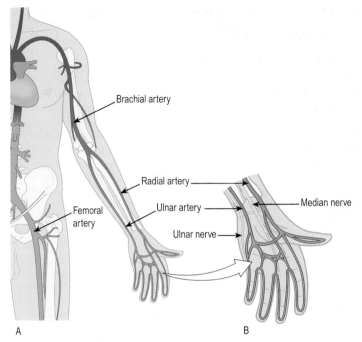

Figure 18 *Arterial puncture sites.*

Box 1.6.1 Contraindications to ABG analysis*

Inadequate collateral circulation at the puncture site

Should not be performed through a lesion or a surgical shunt

Evidence of peripheral vascular disease distant to the puncture site

A coagulopathy or medium- to high-dose anticoagulation therapy

---

*These are not absolute and depend upon the clinical importance of ABG analysis.

RADIAL ARTERY SAMPLING

- Perform a modified Allen test to ensure adequate collateral circulation from ulnar artery[1] (Figure 20).

- Position the patient's hand as shown in Figure 19 with the wrist extended 20–30°. Greater extension of the wrist may impede arterial flow.

- Identify the radial artery by palpating the pulse; choose a site where the pulse is prominent.

- Clean the sampling site with an alcohol wipe.

- Expel the heparin from syringe.

- Steady your hand on the patient's hand, as shown, then insert the needle at 45°, bevel facing up.

- Be sure to insert the needle slowly to minimise the risk of arterial spasm.

- When the needle is in the artery a flash of pulsatile blood will appear in the barrel of the needle. Most ABG syringes will then fill under arterial pressure (see info box over page).

- Obtain at least 3 mL of blood before withdrawing.

---

[1] However, the value of routinely performing a modified Allen's test prior to arterial puncture has been questioned, in part due to its poor sensitivity and specificity for identifying inadequate collateral circulation. (Slogoff S, Keats AS, Arlund C. On the safety of radial artery cannulation. Anaesthesiology 1983;59:42–47).

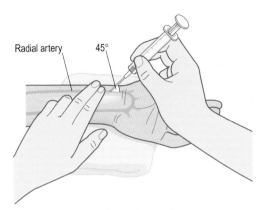

Figure 19 *Positioning of wrist for ABG sampling.*

Tip: local anaesthetic

Arterial sampling (particularly from the radial artery) can be extremely painful; discomfort can be reduced by injecting 1 mL of 1% lidocaine, at the needle insertion site prior to sampling.

Venous or arterial blood?

Dark, non-pulsatile blood that requires manual suction to aspirate often indicates a venous sample (except in severe shock/cardiac arrest). Another clue is when Sao_2 on ABG analysis is significantly lower than Sao_2 on pulse oximetry.

AFTER SAMPLING

- Once adequate blood has been obtained, remove the needle and apply firm, direct pressure to the sample site for at least 5 minutes (and until bleeding has ceased).

- Dispose of all sharps and contaminated materials appropriately.

- Ensure that no air bubbles are present in the sample, as they may compromise results. Any sample with more than very fine bubbles should be discarded.

- The sample should be analysed promptly: if the transit time is likely to exceed 10 minutes, then the syringe should be stored on crushed ice.

- If sampling is unsuccessful it is often advisable to repeat the test on the opposite wrist as even slight irritation of the artery on the first attempt may have provoked arterial spasm, thwarting further attempts at puncture.

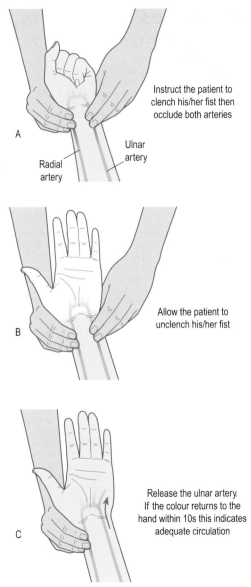

A — Instruct the patient to clench his/her fist then occlude both arteries

Radial artery

Ulnar artery

B — Allow the patient to unclench his/her fist

C — Release the ulnar artery. If the colour returns to the hand within 10s this indicates adequate circulation

Figure 20 *Modified Allen test.*

WHEN AND WHY IS AN ABG REQUIRED?

1. TO ESTABLISH A DIAGNOSIS

The ABG is integral to the diagnosis of respiratory failure and primary hyperventilation. It also identifies the presence of metabolic acidosis and alkalosis.

2. TO ASSESS ILLNESS SEVERITY

The four ABG values shown in the table below, *in addition to overall clinical assessment*, may help identify critically unwell patients requiring urgent intervention.

Pao_2 < 8 kPa
Below 8 kPa, falls in Pao_2 produce a marked reduction in Sao_2 (the 'steep' part of the O_2 dissociation curve) and hence O_2 content of blood
Rising $Paco_2$
Since renal compensation occurs over days to weeks, acute rises in $Paco_2$ produce a corresponding drop in pH. In respiratory distress, rising $Paco_2$ often signifies exhaustion and is an ominous sign. Patients require urgent reversal of the process, leading to ventilatory failure or assisted ventilation
BE < −10/HCO_3 < 15
This value is included in several severity scoring systems and, when due to lactic acidosis, indicates severe hypoxia at cellular level
H+ > 55/pH < 7.25
A significant decrease in pH outside the normal range indicates that compensatory mechanisms have been overwhelmed and is a medical emergency

3. TO GUIDE AND MONITOR TREATMENT

Regular ABG monitoring can help provide early warning of deterioration and judge the effectiveness of therapeutic interventions. It is essential for titrating O_2 therapy in patients with chronic type 2 respiratory failure and for optimising ventilator settings.

Box 1.7.1   Clinical scenarios in which an ABG is useful

Establishing diagnosis and assessing illness severity

Suspected hypercapnia ($\uparrow Pa\text{CO}_2$)
    Drowsiness, flapping tremor, bounding pulses
    Clinical deterioration in patient with chronic type 2 respiratory
    impairment or predisposing condition (e.g. chronic obstructive
    pulmonary disease)
Suspected severe hypoxaemia
    Very low or unrecordable O_2 saturation; cyanosis
Severe, prolonged or worsening respiratory distress
Smoke inhalation (carboxyhaemoglobin level)
Hyperventilation (confirm $\downarrow Pa\text{CO}_2$, check for underlying metabolic acidosis)
Acute deterioration in consciousness
Any severely unwell patient*
Pulse oximetry unreliable or suspicious result
As part of a recognised illness severity scoring system (e.g. Glasgow
criteria in pancreatitis)

Guiding treatment and monitoring response

Mechanically ventilated patients
Patients receiving non-invasive assisted ventilation
Patients with respiratory failure
Patients with chronic hypercapnia receiving O_2
Critically ill patients undergoing surgery
Candidates for long-term oxygen therapy

*Including, but not restricted to, shock, sepsis, burns, major trauma, acute abdomen, poisoning, cardiac/renal/hepatic failure, diabetic ketoacidosis.

COMMON ABG VALUES

The following parameters are commonly found on ABG reports and are provided for reference (normal ranges in brackets):

H^+ (35–45 nmol/L) < 35 = alkalaemia, > 45 = acidaemia

Concentration of free hydrogen ions: this is a measure of how acidic or alkaline a solution is.

pH (7.35–7.45) < 7.35 = acidaemia, > 7.45 = alkalaemia

Negative log of the H^+ ion concentration: this is a common representation of the H^+ concentration. Due to the logarithmic nature of the scale, small changes in the pH actually represent large changes in the H^+ concentration.

P_{O_2} (> 10.6 kPa or > 80 mmHg in arterial blood on room air)

Partial pressure of O_2: can be thought of as the drive for O_2 molecules to move from one place to another. P_{O_2} is not a measure of O_2 content but it does determine the extent to which Hb is saturated with O_2. Pa_{O_2} refers *specifically* to the partial pressure of O_2 in *arterial blood*.

P_{CO_2} (4.7–6.0 kPa or 35–45 mmHg in arterial blood)

Partial pressure of CO_2: can be thought of as the drive for CO_2 molecules to move from one place to another and (unlike P_{O_2}) is directly proportional to the amount of CO_2 in blood. Pa_{CO_2} refers *specifically* to the partial pressure of CO_2 in *arterial blood*.

S_{O_2} (> 96% on room air)

O_2 saturation of haemoglobin: the percentage of O_2-binding sites on Hb proteins occupied by O_2 molecules. This is a measure of how much of the blood's O_2-carrying capacity is being used. Sa_{O_2} refers *specifically* to the O_2 saturation of *arterial blood*.

HCO_3act (22–28 mmol/L)

Actual bicarbonate: the plasma bicarbonate concentration *calculated from* the actual PCO2 and pH measurements in the arterial blood sample. High bicarbonate levels signify a metabolic alkalosis and low levels signify a metabolic acidosis.

HCO_3st (22–28 mmol/L)

Standard bicarbonate: the plasma bicarbonate concentration *calculated from* the PCO2 and pH measurements in the arterial blood sample after the pCO2 in the sample has been corrected to 5.3 KPa (40 mmHg). The authors recommend using this measurement of bicarbonate in ABG analysis.

BE (−2 to +2)

Base excess: a calculation of the amount of base that needs to be added to, or removed from, a sample of blood to achieve a neutral pH, at 37°, *after PCO_2 has been corrected to 5.3 KPa (40 mmHg)*. A positive BE indicates that there is more base than normal (metabolic alkalosis) and a negative BE indicates that there is less base than normal (metabolic acidosis).

Lactate (0.4–1.5 mmol/L)

An indirect measure of lactic acid: high levels of lactic acid are a sign of tissue hypoxia.

Hb (13–18 g/dL men, 11.5–16 g/dL women)

Plasma haemoglobin concentration: this effectively determines blood's capacity to carry O_2.

Na (135–145 mmol/L) Plasma sodium concentration.

K (3.5–5 mmol/L) Plasma potassium concentration.

Cl (95–105 mmol/L) Plasma chloride concentration.

iCa (1.0–1.25 mmol/L) Plasma ionised calcium concentration.

Glucose (3.5–5.5 mmol/L if fasting) Plasma glucose concentration.

MAKING ABG INTERPRETATION EASY

The golden rule for making ABG interpretation easy is to assess pulmonary gas exchange and acid base status *independently*.

ASSESSING PULMONARY GAS EXCHANGE

- Using the algorithm opposite, classify gas exchange into one of the four possible categories.

- If there is type 1 respiratory impairment, assess severity of hypoxaemia (box 1)

- If there is type 2 respiratory impairment, establish whether it is chronic or acute, then assess severity of hypercapnia and hypoxaemia (boxes 1 & 2)

- If the category is hyperventilation, determine whether it is primary or secondary.

Table 1.9.1 Assessing hypoxaemia severity

	Pao_2	Sao_2
Mild	8–10.6 kPa 60–79 mmHg	90–94%
Moderate	5.3–7.9 kPa 40–59 mmHg	75–89%
Severe	< 5.3 kPa < 40 mmHg or: High FiO_2 requirements to maintain adequate Pao_2	< 75%

Box 1.9.1 Assessing hypercapnia severity

Severity is not related to absolute $Paco_2$ value but to the *rate of $Paco_2$ rise* and degree of blood pH derangement (pH < 7.25 = severe acidaemia). The presence of exhaustion is also an ominous sign.

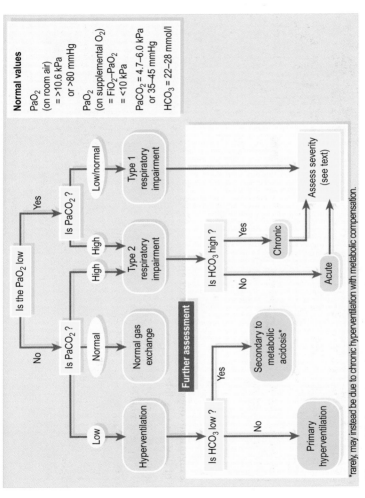

Normal values

PaO_2
(on room air)
= >10.6 kPa
or >80 mmHg

PaO_2
(on supplemental O_2)
= FiO_2–PaO_2
= <10 kPa

$PaCO_2$ = 4.7–6.0 kPa
or 35–45 mmHg

HCO_3 = 22–28 mmol/l

Is the PaO_2 low

No — Yes

Is $PaCO_2$?

Low — Hyperventilation

Normal — Normal gas exchange

High — Type 2 respiratory impairment

Is $PaCO_2$?

High — Type 2 respiratory impairment

Low/normal — Type 1 respiratory impairment

Further assessment

Is HCO_3 low ?

Yes — Secondary to metabolic acidosis*

No — Primary hyperventilation

Is HCO_3 high ?

Yes — Chronic

No — Acute

Chronic → Assess severity (see text)

Acute → Assess severity (see text)

Type 1 respiratory impairment → Assess severity (see text)

*rarely, may instead be due to chronic hyperventilation with metabolic compensation.

Figure 21 *Assessing pulmonary gas exchange.*

INTERPRETING ACID-BASE STATUS

- Use the flow chart opposite to broadly classify acid-base status.
- If the patient has a metabolic acidosis, calculate the anion gap to narrow down the differential diagnosis.

  Anion Gap = $(Na + K) - (Cl + HCO_3)$ Normal = $10 - 18$ mmol/l

- If the precise acid-base derangement is not immediately clear (e.g. middle column) then remember the following points:

  Always consider the clinical context when interpreting acid-base status.

  Metabolic compensation takes days to occur, respiratory compensation takes minutes.

  Overcompensation does not occur.

  An apparent compensatory response could represent an opposing primary process.

- Note that with a very mild acidaemia or alkalaemia both $PaCO_2$ and HCO_3 may be just within the "normal range" (considered to be a mild mixed acid-base disturbance).

Normal values

$PaCO_2 = 4.7 – 6.0$ kPa or $35 – 45$ mmHg

BE (−2 to +2)

HCO_3 st (22–28 mmol/l)

pH (7.35–7.45)

H^+ (35–45 nmol/l)

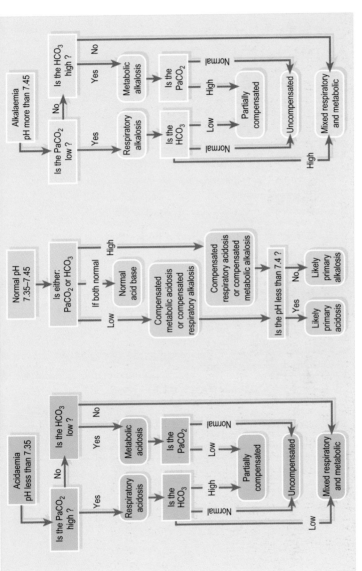

Figure 22 *Acid–base status.*

APPENDIX 1

A–a gradient

The A–a gradient is the difference between the P_{O_2} in alveoli (PA_{O_2}) and the P_{O_2} in arterial blood (Pa_{O_2}). Pa_{O_2} is measured on ABG but PA_{O_2} has to be calculated using the alveolar gas equation (see box below).

$$A - a\ gradient = PA_{O_2} - Pa_{O_2}$$

It is normally less than 2.6 kPa (20 mmHg), although it increases with age and FiO_2. This means that:

1. the normal range for Pa_{O_2} falls with age
2. the A–a gradient is most accurate when performed on room air

---

Simplified alveolar gas equation*

$$PA_{O_2}\ (kPa) = (FiO_2 \times 93.8) - (Pa_{CO_2} \times 1.2)$$

or

$$PA_{O_2}\ (mmHg) = (FiO_2 \times 713) - (Pa_{CO_2} \times 1.2)$$

*Assumes the patient is at sea level and has a body temperature of 37°C.

PART 2

THE ABG IN PRACTICE

CASE 1

History

A 25-year-old man, with no significant past medical history, presents to the emergency department with a 2-day history of fever, productive cough and worsening breathlessness.

Examination

He is hot and flushed with a temperature of 39.3°C. He does not appear distressed but is using accessory muscles of respiration. There is diminished chest expansion on the left with dullness to percussion, bronchial breathing and coarse crackles in the left lower zone posteriorly.

Pulse	104 beats/min
Respiratory rate	28 breaths/min
Blood pressure	118/70 mmHg
SaO_2 (room air)	89%

Arterial blood gas	**On room air**	
23/7/2006		
Unit no.: 00654545		
ID: John Simpson	Normal	
H$^+$	31.8 nmol/L	(35–45)
pH	7.50	(7.35–7.45)
PCO_2	3.74 kPa	(4.7–6.0)
	28.1 mmHg	(35–45)
PO_2	7.68 kPa	(> 10.6)
	57.8 mmHg	(> 80)
Bicarb	23.9 mmol/L	(22–28)
BE	–0.5 mmol/L	(–2–+2)
SPO_2	88.7%	(> 98%)
Lactate	1.2	(0.4–1.5)
K	3.7 mmol/L	(3.5–5)
Na	138 mmol/L	(135–145)
Cl	99 mmol/L	(95–105)
iCa$^+$	1.2 mmol/L	(1–1.25)
Hb	15 g/dL	(13–18)
Glucose	5.4 mmol/L	(3.5–5.5)

Questions

1. a) Describe his gas exchange.
   b) Describe his acid–base status.

2. Should the patient receive supplemental O$_2$?

3. Is pulse oximetry a suitable alternative to repeated ABG monitoring in this case?

CASE 2

History

A 34-year-old morbidly obese female with a body mass index of 49 has an ABG sample taken as part of her preoperative assessment for weight reduction surgery.

Apart from morbid obesity and type 2 diabetes, she is otherwise well and has no respiratory symptoms.

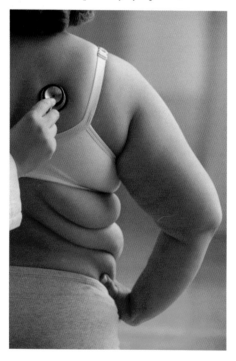

Arterial blood gas	**On air**	
14/01/2005		
Unit no.: 55392088		
ID: Marcella Plantagenet		
		Normal
H^+	45 nmol/L	(35–45)
pH	7.35	(7.35–7.45)
P_{CO_2}	7.3 kPa	(4.7–6.0)
	54.8 mmHg	(35–45)
P_{O_2}	9.6 kPa	(> 10.6)
	72.2 mmHg	(> 80)
Bicarb	29 mmol/L	(22–28)
BE	+3.8	(–2–+2)
S_{PO_2}	96%	(> 98%)
Lactate	1	(0.4 – 1.5)
K	4.7 mmol/L	(3.5–5)
Na	134 mmol/L	(135–145)
Cl	102 mmol/L	(95–105)
iCa^+	1.2 mmol/L	(1–1.25)
Hb	13 g/dL	(13–18)
Glucose	9 mmol/L	(3.5–5.5)

Questions

1. a) Describe her gas exchange.
   b) Describe her acid–base status.

2. What is the most likely diagnosis?

CASE 3

History

A 24-year-old female nursing student attends hospital complaining of sudden-onset breathlessness. She flew to the UK from Australia the previous day and is very concerned she may have a pulmonary embolism. She has no pleuritic pain, haemoptysis or leg swelling, no past history of lung disease or deep-vein thrombosis and is a non-smoker.

Examination

She appears anxious and distressed. Her respiratory rate is elevated but chest examination is unremarkable and there are no clinical signs of deep-vein thrombosis. A chest X-ray reveals no abnormalities.

Pulse	88 beats/min
Respiratory rate	22 breaths/min
Blood pressure	124/76 mmHg
SaO_2 (room air)	95%

23/7/2006
Unit no.: 00654545
ID: Jill Royds

		Normal
H⁺	31.2 nmol/L	(35–45)
pH	7.51	(7.35–7.45)
P_{CO_2}	3.90 kPa	(4.7–6.0)
	29.3 mmHg	(35–45)
P_{O_2}	10.3 kPa	(> 10.6)
	77.0 mmHg	(> 80)
Bicarb	25.0 mmol/L	(22–28)
BE	+0.7 mmol/L	(−2–+2)
Sp_{O_2}	93.7%	(> 98%)
Lactate	1.0	(0.4 – 1.5)
K	4.3 mmol/L	(3.5–5)
Na	141 mmol/L	(135–145)
Cl	101 mmol/L	(95–105)
iCa⁺	1.2 mmol/L	(1–1.25)
Hb	13 g/dL	(13–18)
Glucose	4.6 mmol/L	(3.5–5.5)

Questions

1. a) Describe her gas exchange.
   b) Describe her acid–base status.

2. What is the likeliest diagnosis?

CASE 4

History

A 78-year-old male on a surgical ward is found unresponsive, having returned, a few hours previously, from a complicated open cholecystectomy.

Review of his charts reveals he has received three 10 mg injections of morphine since returning to the ward, in addition to the morphine delivered by his patient-controlled analgesia device.

Examination

The patient is unresponsive with shallow respirations and bilateral pinpoint pupils.

Pulse rate	90 beats/min
Respiratory rate	5 breaths/min
Blood pressure	98/64 mmHg
SaO_2	99%
BM	5.6 mmol/l

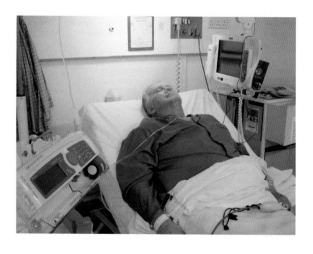

Arterial blood gas		**On 28% O$_2$**
18/09/2006		
Unit no.: 6799986		
ID: Henry Spasek		
		Normal
H$^+$	65.4 nmol/L	(35–45)
pH	7.18	(7.35–7.45)
PCO$_2$	8.2 kPa	(4.7–6.0)
	62 mmHg	(35–45)
PO$_2$	11.76 kPa	(> 10.6)
	87 mmHg	(> 80)
Bicarb	22.4 mmol/L	(22–28)
BE	–1.5 mmol/L	(–2–+2)
SPO$_2$	99.8%	(> 98%)
Lactate	1	(0.4–1.5)
K	4.4 mmol/L	(3.5–5)
Na	137 mmol/L	(135–145)
Cl	103 mmol/L	(95–105)
iCa$^+$	1.16 mmol/L	(1–1.25)
Hb	11 g/dL	(13–18)
Glucose	3.9 mmol/L	(3.5–5.5)

Questions

1. a) Describe his gas exchange.
   b) Describe his acid–base status.

2. What is the most likely diagnosis?

3. What treatment does this patient require?

CASE 5

History

A 75-year-old man is brought into the emergency department by his family. He is extremely short of breath and struggling to speak.

Following a conversation with his family it emerges that he has a long history of chronic obstructive pulmonary disease.

Over the last 3 days his breathing has worsened considerably and he has expectorated increased volumes of sputum.

Examination

The patient is struggling for breath and appears extremely distressed. He exhibits signs of chest hyperinflation and is breathing through pursed lips. Breath sounds are generally diminished but there are no added sounds.

Pulse	120 beats/min
Respiratory rate	26 breaths/min
Blood pressure	150/80 mmHg
Temperature	36°C
$SaO_2\%$	81%

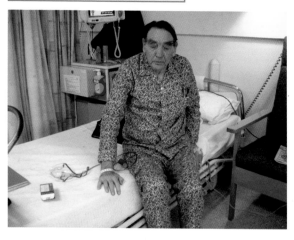

Arterial blood gas		**On air**
10/07/2005		
Unit no.: 77655349		
ID: Joseph Spielman		
		Normal
H$^+$	39.5 nmol/L	(35–45)
pH	7.40	(7.35–7.45)
P_{CO_2}	4.9 kPa	(4.7–6.0)
	36 mmHg	(35–45)
P_{O_2}	5.8 kPa	(> 10.6)
	44 mmHg	(> 80)
Bicarb	23 mmol/L	(22–28)
BE	–1.2 mmol/L	(–2–+2)
SP_{O_2}	80%	(> 98%)
Lactate	1.0	(0.4–1.5)
K	4.1 mmol/L	(3.5–5)
Na	137 mmol/L	(135–145)
Cl	99 mmol/L	(95–105)
iCa$^+$	1.1 mmol/L	(1–1.25)
Hb	16.5 g/dL	(13–18)
Glucose	3.8 mmol/L	(3.5–5.5)

Questions

1. a) Describe his gas exchange.

b) Describe his acid–base status.

2. Should you provide him with oxygen?

CASE 6

History

The patient from the previous case is treated in the emergency department with nebulised bronchodilators, oral prednisolone and antibiotics. He is then transferred to a respiratory ward where he is administered 28% oxygen by a fixed concentration mask. Despite this, his SaO_2 (as measured by pulse oximetry) increases only marginally and there is no improvement in his symptoms.

Examination

Examination findings in the chest are unchanged but he now appears exhausted and slightly confused.

Pulse	120 beats/min
Respiratory rate	16 breaths/min
Blood pressure	120/80 mmHg
SaO_2	83% (on 28% O_2)
Temperature	36°C

A repeat ABG is performed (6 hours after the first ABG).

Arterial blood gas		**On 28% O$_2$**
11/07/2005		
Unit no.: 77655349		
ID: Joseph Spielman		
		Normal
H$^+$	51.4 nmol/L	(35–45)
pH	7.29	(7.35–7.45)
PCO$_2$	6.9 kPa	(4.7–6.0)
	52 mmHg	(35–45)
PO$_2$	6.4 kPa	(> 10.6)
	48 mmHg	(> 80)
Bicarb	24 mmol/L	(22–28)
BE	–0.9 mmol/L	(–2–+2)
SPO$_2$	84%	(> 98%)
Lactate	1.0	(0.4–1.5)
K	4.0 mmol/L	(3.5–5)
Na	137 mmol/L	(135–145)
Cl	99 mmol/L	(95–105)
iCa$^+$	1.1 mmol/L	(1–1.25)
Hb	16.5 g/dL	(13–18)
Glucose	4.2 mmol/L	(3.5–5.5)

Questions

1. a) Describe his gas exchange.
   b) Describe his acid–base status.

2. Should his oxygen now be stopped?

CASE 7

History

A 77-year-old woman is admitted to the stroke ward with right-sided weakness, visual disturbance and slurred speech. She is commenced on nasogastric feeding due to swallowing problems but has a large vomit 24 hours later. She initially appears well but over the next few hours develops worsening breathing difficulties.

Examination

She is agitated, distressed and pyrexial. A dull percussion note and coarse crackles are evident at both lung bases. Other than acute confusion, neurological findings are unchanged from admission.

Pulse	92 beats/min
Respiratory rate	28 breaths/min
Blood pressure	112/65 mmHg
SaO_2 (60% O_2)	92%

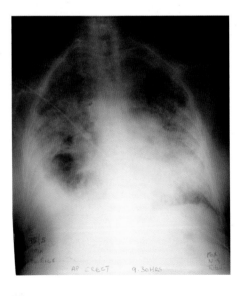

Arterial blood gas		**On 60% O$_2$**
23/7/2006		
Unit no.: 00654545		
ID: Mary Waters		
		Normal
H$^+$	38.8 nmol/L	(35–45)
pH	7.41	(7.35–7.45)
Pco_2	4.43 kPa	(4.7–6.0)
	33.2 mmHg	(35–45)
Po_2	8.67 kPa	(> 10.6)
	65.0 mmHg	(> 80)
Bicarb	21.2 mmol/L	(22–28)
BE	–2.8 mmol/L	(–2–+2)
Spo_2	92.7%	(> 98%)
Lactate	1.6	(0.4–1.5)
K	4.0 mmol/L	(3.5–5)
Na	144 mmol/L	(135–145)
Cl	103 mmol/L	(95–105)
iCa$^+$	1.2 mmol/L	(1–1.25)
Hb	13 g/dL	(13–18)
Glucose	6.6 mmol/L	(3.5–5.5)

Questions

1. a) Describe her gas exchange.
   b) Describe her acid–base status.

2. What is the most likely diagnosis?

3. Is her condition mild, moderate or severe?

CASE 8

History

A 68-year-old man with chronic obstructive pulmonary disease is referred to hospital by his doctor with a short history of increased breathlessness and reduced effort tolerance. He is normally capable of walking around 500 metres but now has difficulty dressing and is breathless at rest.

Examination

He is lucid, alert and mildly distressed. He is using accessory muscles of respiration and breathing through pursed lips. Chest examination reveals features of hyperinflation, generally diminished breath sounds and scattered rhonchi (wheeze).

Pulse	96 beats/min
Respiratory rate	24 breaths/min
Blood pressure	138/82 mmHg
SaO_2 (room air)	78%

Arterial blood gas		**On air**
23/7/2006		
Unit no.: 00654545		
ID: Hamish Roy		
		Normal
H^+	43.2 nmol/L	(35–45)
pH	7.36	(7.35–7.45)
P_{CO_2}	7.20 kPa	(4.7–6.0)
	54.1 mmHg	(35–45)
P_{O_2}	5.3 kPa	(> 10.6)
	40 mmHg	(> 80)
Bicarb	30.6 mmol/L	(22–28)
BE	+4.9 mmol/L	(–2–+2)
SP_{O_2}	75.2%	(> 98%)
Lactate	1.2	(0.4–1.5)
K	3.7 mmol/L	(3.5–5)
Na	144 mmol/L	(135–145)
Cl	102 mmol/L	(95–105)
iCa^+	1.2 mmol/L	(1–1.25)
Hb	16 g/dL	(13–18)
Glucose	4.9 mmol/L	(3.5–5.5)

Questions

1. a) Describe his gas exchange.
   b) Describe his acid–base status.

2. Which one of the following ABG values is most likely to have changed significantly in the past 24 hours: pH, PCO_2, PO_2 or HCO_3?

3. Which two of the above ABG values indicate the need for caution when providing O_2 therapy?

CASE 9

History

The patient from the previous case is treated with nebulised bronchodilators, oral prednisolone and 60% O_2 by face mask. His oxygen saturations improve significantly but when he is reviewed 1 hour later, his condition has deteriorated and he is unable to provide a history.

Examination

He is drowsy and barely rousable. He no longer appears to be in respiratory distress and his respiratory rate has fallen to 14 breaths/min. Chest examination is unchanged from previously.

Pulse	88 beats/min
Respiratory rate	14 breaths/min
Blood pressure	132/80 mmHg
SaO_2 (room air)	96%

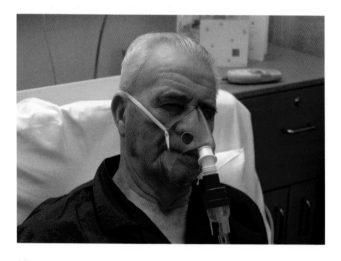

Arterial blood gas		**On 60% O$_2$**
23/7/2006		
Unit no.: 00654545		
ID: Hamish Roy		
		Normal
H$^+$	50.8 nmol/L	(35–45)
pH	7.29	(7.35–7.45)
P$_{CO_2}$	8.7 kPa	(4.7–6.0)
	65.3 mmHg	(35–45)
P$_{O_2}$	11.2 kPa	(> 10.6)
	84.0 mmHg	(> 80)
Bicarb	30.3 mmol/L	(24–30)
BE	+4.7 mmol/L	(–2–+2)
S$_{PO_2}$	96.2%	(> 98%)
Lactate	1.2	(0.4–1.5)
K	3.6 mmol/L	(3.5–5)
Na	144 mmol/L	(135–145)
Cl	102 mmol/L	(95–105)
iCa$^+$	1.2 mmol/L	(1–1.25)
Hb	16 g/dL	(13–18)
Glucose	5.0 mmol/L	(3.5–5.5)

Questions

1. a) Describe his gas exchange.

   b) Describe his acid–base status.

2. What has been the cause of his deterioration?

CASE 10

History

A 21-year-old woman presents to the emergency department with a 6-hour history of worsening breathlessness and wheeze. She has a past history of asthma with two previous exacerbations requiring hospital admission. She now feels very breathless and is obtaining no relief from her salbutamol inhaler.

Examination

She is tachypnoeic at 30 breaths/min, is using her accessory muscles of respiration and only just managing to speak in full sentences.

Auscultation of her chest reveals widespread polyphonic wheeze.

Pulse	115 beats/min
Blood pressure	120/80 mmHg
SpO_2	96% (room air)
Peak expiratory flow	160 L/s (predicted = 400 L/s)

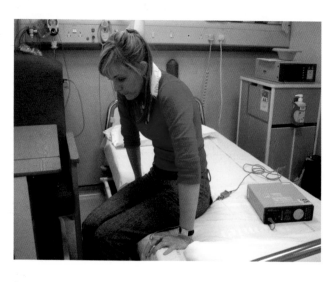

Arterial blood gas 12/11/2005 Unit no.: 12639943 ID: Jessica Goldman	**On air**	
		Normal
H^+	42 nmol/L	(35–45)
pH	7.38	(7.35–7.45)
P_{CO_2}	5.8 kPa	(4.7–6.0)
	43 mmHg	(35–45)
P_{O_2}	10.2 kPa	(> 10.6)
	76 mmHg	(> 80)
Bicarb	24 mmol/L	(22–28)
BE	–1.3 mmol/L	(–2–+2)
Sa_{O_2}	96%	(> 98%)
Lactate	1	(0.4 – 1.5)
K	4.0 mmol/L	(3.5–5)
Na	140 mmol/L	(135–145)
Cl	99 mmol/L	(95–105)
iCa^+	1.12 mmol/L	(1–1.25)
Hb	13.0 g/dL	(11.5–15.5)
Glucose	5 mmol/L	(3.5–5.5)

Questions

1. a) Describe her gas exchange.
   b) Describe her acid–base status.

2. Which of the above ABG values gives the greatest cause for concern?

3. How would you classify the severity of this asthma attack?

CASE 11

History

A 23-year-old woman presents to the emergency department with a painful ankle, following a simple trip. While being examined by the emergency department doctor she becomes extremely agitated and upset. Despite a normal ankle X-ray and extensive reassurance by the emergency department staff, she refuses to believe that her ankle is not broken and starts crying. While leaving the department, she develops a clutching sensation in her chest, shortness of breath and a tingling sensation in her hands and around her mouth. She reports that she feels unable to take a deep breath.

Examination

The patient appears frightened and extremely distressed. Other than tachypnoea and a mild sinus tachycardia, cardiorespiratory examination is unremarkable. Electrocardiogram, chest X-ray and peak flow measurements are all normal.

Pulse	96 beats/min
Respiratory rate	36 breaths/min
Blood pressure	130/80 mmHg
SpO_2	100%

Arterial blood gas 12/11/2006 Unit no.: 12534943 ID: Trinny Farqhuar	**On air**	
		Normal
H⁺	29 nmol/L	(35–45)
pH	7.53	(7.35–7.45)
P_{CO_2}	3.14 kPa	(4.7–6.0)
	24 mmHg	(35–45)
P_{O_2}	14.3 kPa	(> 10.6)
	108 mmHg	(> 80)
Bicarb	24 mmol/L	(22–28)
BE	–1.8 mmol/L	(–2–+2)
Sa_{O_2}	99%	(> 98%)
Lactate	1	(0.4–1.5)
K	3.5 mmol/L	(3.5–5)
Na	140 mmol/L	(135–145)
Cl	99 mmol/L	(95–105)
iCa⁺	0.9 mmol/L	(1–1.25)
Hb	12.0 g/dL	(11.5–15.5)
Glucose	5 mmol/L	(3.5–5.5)

Questions

1. a) Describe her gas exchange.

b) Describe her acid–base status.

2. Are there any other abnormalities?

3. What is the likely diagnosis?

CASE 12

History

A 40-year-old male is pulled from a house fire and brought to the emergency department in the early hours of the morning. The paramedics estimate he is likely to have been trapped in a smoke-filled room for up to 20 minutes prior to rescue.

Examination

The patient is heavily contaminated with soot and smells strongly of smoke. Fortunately he has not sustained any thermal injuries. He appears to be confused and has just vomited.

Baseline observations are normal, with an oxygen saturation of 99% on 15 L O_2 by mask.

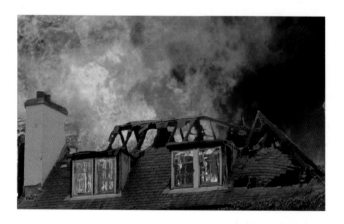

Arterial blood gas		**On 15 L O$_2$ by mask**
10/08/2005		
Unit no.: 77634566		
ID: Robert Jones		
		Normal
H$^+$	44 nmol/L	(35–45)
pH	7.36	(7.35–7.45)
PCO$_2$	4.5 kPa	(4.7–6.0)
	34 mmHg	(35–45)
PO$_2$	47 kPa	(> 10.6)
	353 mmHg	(> 80)
Bicarb	18 mmol/L	(22–28)
BE	–5.5 mmol/L	(–2–+2)
SPO$_2$	100%	(> 98%)
Lactate	2	(0.4–1.5)
K	3.6 mmol/L	(3.5–5)
Na	145 mmol/L	(135–145)
Cl	103 mmol/L	(95–105)
iCa$^+$	1.1 mmol/L	(1–1.25)
Hb	14 g/dL	(13–18)
Glucose	4 mmol/L	(3.5–5.5)

Carbon monoxide assay

CO	40%	(non-smokers < 3%)
		(smokers < 10%)

Questions

1. a) Describe his gas exchange.

b) Describe his acid–base status.

2. What is the most likely diagnosis?

3. Which of the values provided is *falsely high*: PaO$_2$, SaO$_2$ or Hb?

CASE 13

History

A 79-year-old female has just been admitted to the general surgical ward to have a large bowel tumour surgically removed.

The tumour was discovered at colonoscopy after she presented to her doctor with a six month history of rectal bleeding.

On admission she appears to be severely short of breath and extremely tired. Further questioning reveals that her rectal blood loss has been no greater than usual.

Pulse	100 beats/min
Blood pressure	100/80 mmHg
Respiratory rate	24 breaths/min
$SaO_2\%$ (on air)	100%

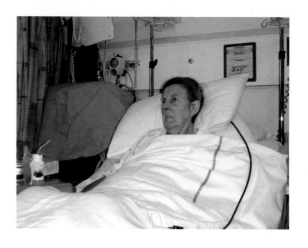

Arterial blood gas	**On air**	
06/06/2005		
Unit no.: 943778		
ID: Ethyl Swainson		
		Normal
H^+	32.3 nmol/L	(35–45)
pH	7.49	(7.35–7.45)
PCO_2	3.31 kPa	(4.7–6.0)
	25 mmHg	(35–45)
PO_2	11.9 kPa	(> 10.6)
	89 mmHg	(> 80)
Bicarb	22 mmol/L	(22–28)
BE	–2 mmol/L	(–2–+2)
SPO_2	99.8%	(> 98%)
Lactate	1	(0.4–1.5)
K	3.8 mmol/L	(3.5–5)
Na	138 mmol/L	(135–145)
Cl	96 mmol/L	(95–105)
iCa^+	1.17 mmol/L	(1–1.25)
Hb	6.8 g/dL	(13–18)
Glucose	3.9 mmol/L	(3.5–5.5)

Questions

1. a) Describe her gas exchange?
   b) Describe her acid-base state?

2. What is the most likely cause of her breathlessness?

3. What would be the most effective way of improving O_2 delivery to her tissues?

CASE 14

History

A 78-year-old woman is admitted to the emergency department with sudden-onset, generalised, severe, abdominal pain. She describes the pain as being colicky with no particular radiation. She does not complain of any alteration in her bowel habit, and has not vomited. Her only medical history is that of atrial fibrillation, for which she takes aspirin and digoxin.

Examination

On examination, the patient is haemodynamically stable with warm, well-perfused peripheries. Despite severe abdominal discomfort, abdominal examination is relatively unremarkable: the abdomen is soft in all four quadrants and is only tender on deep palpation. No hernias or aneurysms are palpable and rectal examination is unremarkable.

An abdominal and erect chest X-ray are taken and found to be normal.

During the course of the examination her clinical condition deteriorates and she is moved to the resuscitation area.

Arterial blood gas **On 10 L O$_2$ by mask**
10/08/2006
Unit no.: 7734211
ID: Susan Ulrik

		Normal
H$^+$	52.5nmol/L	(35–45)
pH	7.28	(7.35–7.45)
P$_{CO_2}$	4.39 kPa	(4.7–6.0)
	33 mmHg	(35–45)
P$_{O_2}$	28.6 kPa	(> 10.6)
	215 mmHg	(> 80)
Bicarb	16.2 mmol/L	(22–28)
BE	–10.4 mmol/L	(–2–+2)
S$_{PO_2}$	99.8%	(> 98%)
Lactate	3.2	(0.4–1.5)
K	4.6 mmol/L	(3.5–5)
Na	135 mmol/L	(135–145)
Cl	96 mmol/L	(95–105)
iCa$^+$	1.16 mmol/L	(1–1.25)
Hb	12 g/dL	(13–18)
Glucose	3.8 mmol/L	(3.5–5.5)

Questions

1. a) Describe her gas exchange.
   b) Describe her acid–base status.

2. What is the most likely diagnosis?

CASE 15

History

A 35-year-old woman with type 1 diabetes is brought to the emergency department by ambulance after being found in her house severely unwell. Following a discussion with her partner it emerges she has not been eating for the past few days due to a vomiting illness and, as a precaution, has also been omitting her insulin.

Examination

On examination, she appears drowsy and peripherally shut-down, with very dry mucous membranes. Her breath smells of acetone and her respirations are deep and sighing.

Pulse	130 beats/min
Blood pressure	100/60 mmHg
Respiratory rate	26 breaths/min
BM (blood glucose)	> 25 mmol/L

Physical examination of her chest and abdomen is unremarkable.

Arterial blood gas		**On 10 L O_2 by mask**
27/02/2005		
Unit no.: 77735566		
ID: Isla Tanner		
		Normal
H^+	88.9 nmol/L	(35–45)
pH	7.05	(7.35–7.45)
P_{CO_2}	1.5 kPa	(4.7–6.0)
	11 mmHg	(35–45)
P_{O_2}	28.4 kPa	(> 10.6)
	187 mmHg	(> 80)
Bicarb	6.0 mmol/L	(24–30)
BE	–25.2 mmol/L	(–2–+2)
SP_{O_2}	99.8%	(> 98%)
Lactate	1	(0.4–1.5)
K	4.6 mmol/L	(3.5–5)
Na	141 mmol/L	(135–145)
Cl	96 mmol/L	(95–105)
iCa^+	1.25 mmol/L	(1–1.25)
Hb	12 g/dL	(13–18)
Glucose	35 mmol/L	(3.5–5.5)

Questions

1. a) Describe her gas exchange.
   b) Describe her acid–base status.

2. Calculate the anion gap.

3. What is the most likely diagnosis?

CASE 16

History

A 37-year-old well-known local vagrant is brought into the department unconscious. He was found near a bottle of vodka and a half-empty bottle of what appears to be methanol. It is unclear if he has drunk any of the contents.

Examination

The patient is unkempt with a significantly reduced conscious level (Glasgow coma scale score = 9). There are no apparent focal neurological abnormalities.

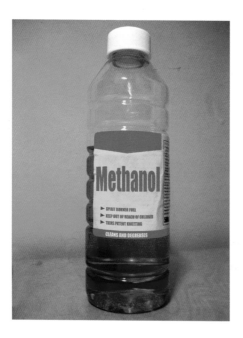

Arterial blood gas		**On air**	
10/07/2006			
Unit no.: 35477899			
ID: Gary Souness			
		Normal	
H$^+$	63.3 nmol/L	(35–45)	
pH	7.20	(7.35–7.45)	
P_{CO_2}	3.3 kPa	(4.7–6.0)	
	25 mmHg	(35–45)	
P_{O_2}	12.8 kPa	(> 10.6)	
	96 mmHg	(> 80)	
Bicarb	9.5 mmol/L	(22–28)	
BE	–16.2 mmol/L	(–2–+2)	
SP_{O_2}	97.8%	(> 98%)	
Lactate	1.3	(0.4–1.5)	
K	4.5 mmol/L	(3.5–5)	
Na	136 mmol/L	(135–145)	
Cl	99 mmol/L	(95–105)	
iCa$^+$	1.1 mmol/L	(1–1.25)	
Hb	13.5 g/dL	(13–18)	
Glucose	3.8 mmol/L	(3.5–5.5)	

Questions

1. a) Describe his gas exchange.
   b) Describe his acid–base status.

2. What is the anion gap?

3. Is the acid–base status consistent with methanol ingestion?

CASE 17

History

A 52-year-old man is being investigated on the urology ward for recurrent renal stones. He also complains of mild fatigue and lethargy. There is no history of gastrointestinal disturbance and he is not on any regular medications.

Examination

The patient is well and clinical examination reveals no abnormalities.

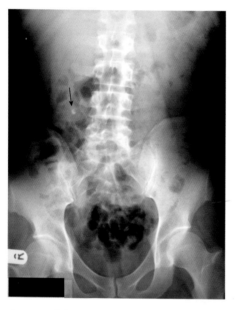

As part of the investigations an ABG is obtained.

Arterial blood gas **On air**
23/04/2006
Unit no.: 27634943
ID: Roger Parry

		Normal
H$^+$	43 nmol/L	(35–45)
pH	7.37	(7.35–7.45)
P_{CO_2}	4.2 kPa	(4.7–6.0)
	31.5 mmHg	(35–45)
P_{O_2}	13.2 kPa	(> 10.6)
	99.0 mmHg	(>80)
Bicarb	18 mmol/L	(22–28)
BE	–7 mmol/L	(–2–+2)
S_{PO_2}	99%	(> 98%)
Lactate	1	(0.4–1.5)
K	3.0 mmol/L	(3.5–5)
Na	137 mmol/L	(135–145)
Cl	109 mmol/L	(95–105)
iCa$^+$	1.0 mmol/L	(1–1.25)
Hb	13.0 g/dL	(11.5–15.5)
Glucose	4 mmol/L	(3.5–5.5)

Questions

1. a) Describe his gas exchange.

   b) Describe his acid–base status.

2. Calculate the anion gap.

3. What is the likeliest diagnosis?

CASE 18

History

An 18-year-old is admitted to the toxicology unit having taken a large overdose of an unknown substance 5 hours earlier. She complains of nausea and a high-pitched noise in her ears.

Examination

On examination, she is mildly confused. Her respirations are increased in both rate and depth. Examination is otherwise unremarkable.

Pulse	100 beats/min
Respiratory rate	26 breaths/min
Blood pressure	132/100 mmHg
Temperature	37.6°C
$O_2\%$	99%

Arterial blood gas	**On air**	
10/09/2006		
Unit no.: 27634943		
ID: Libby Farqhuar		
		Normal
H+	38.8 nmol/L	(35–45)
pH	7.41	(7.35–7.45)
P_{CO_2}	3.01 kPa	(4.7–6.0)
	22.6 mmHg	(35–45)
P_{O_2}	14.1 kPa	(> 10.6)
	97.5 mmHg	(> 80)
Bicarb	17.6 mmol/L	(22–28)
BE	–8.3 mmol/L	(–2–+2)
SP_{O_2}	99%	(> 98%)
Lactate	1.4	(0.4–1.5)
K	3.6 mmol/L	(3.5–5)
Na	140 mmol/L	(135–145)
Cl	99 mmol/L	(95–105)
iCa+	1.2 mmol/L	(1–1.25)
Hb	13.0 g/dL	(11.5–15.5)
Glucose	5 mmol/L	(3.5–5.5)

Questions

1. a) Describe her gas exchange.
   b) Describe her acid–base status.

2. Calculate the anion gap.

3. What substance is she most likely to have taken?

CASE 19

History

A 24 year old man is brought to hospital by his family after becoming unwell at home. They report that he has no history of significant medical illness but has recently been undergoing tests for progressive fatigue and weight loss. Over the last few days he has become increasingly weak and lethargic and has also complained of muscle cramps. They became alarmed today when he appeared drowsy and disoriented.

Examination

The patient appears listless and confused. He has cool peripheries and poor capillary refill. He is afebrile and there is no rash, lymphadenopathy or meningism. Abdominal examination is unremarkable and there are no focal chest or neurological signs.

Pulse	120 beats/min
Respiratory rate	25 breaths/min
Blood pressure	75/55 mmHg
Temperature	36.5°C
BM	2.9

Arterial blood gas	**On air**	
10/08/2005		
Unit no.: 456986793		
ID: Rufus Wainwright		
		Normal
H⁺	48 nmol/L	(35–45)
pH	7.32	(7.35–7.45)
P_{CO_2}	3.3 kPa	(4.7–6.0)
	24.8 mmHg	(35–45)
P_{O_2}	13 kPa	(> 10.6)
	97 mmHg	(> 80)
Bicarb	13.4 mmol/L	(22–28)
BE	–13.9 mmol/L	(–2–+2)
S_{O_2}	99%	(> 98%)
Lactate	3	(0.4–1.5)
K	5.6 mmol/L	(3.5–5)
Na	125 mmol/L	(135–145)
Cl	101 mmol/L	(95–105)
iCa⁺	1.2 mmol/L	(1–1.25)
Hb	13.0 g/dL	(13–18)
Glucose	2.5 mmol/L	(3.5–5.5)

Questions

1. a) Describe his gas exchange.
   b) Describe his acid–base state?

2. Are there any other abnormalities on the ABG?

3. What specific treatment does this patient require?

CASE 20

History

An 87-year-old man has been found collapsed in the ward toilet. Cardiopulmonary resuscitation was commenced promptly, as no pulse or respiratory effort was detected, and has now been in progress for 12 minutes. He has a past medical history of ischaemic heart disease, dementia and chronic renal failure.

Examination

The patient has a Glasgow coma scale score of 3 and appears pale and mottled. The cardiac monitor reveals an agonal rhythm as shown below. No pulses are palpable and there is no respiratory effort. He is currently being ventilated by a bag and mask on 15 L/min of O_2.

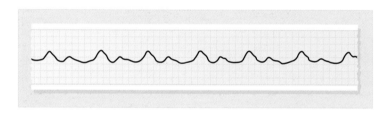

Arterial blood gas 10/02/2004 Unit no.: 42333993 ID: David King		**On 15 L O₂ by bag mask**
		Normal
H⁺	160 nmol/L	(35–45)
pH	6.8	(7.35–7.45)
P_{CO_2}	4.8 kPa	(4.7–6.0)
	36 mmHg	(35–45)
P_{O_2}	32 kPa	(> 10.6)
	240 mmHg	(> 80)
Bicarb	3.8 mmol/L	(22–28)
BE	–20 mmol/L	(–2–+2)
S_{O_2}	100%	(> 98%)
Lactate	9	(0.4–1.5)
K	4.5 mmol/L	(3.5–5)
Na	136 mmol/L	(135–145)
Cl	96 mmol/L	(95–105)
Ca⁺	1.1 mmol/L	(1–1.25)
Hb	14.0 g/dL	(13.5–18.5)
Glucose	4 mmol/L	(3.5–5.5)

Questions

1. a) Describe his gas exchange.
   b) Describe his acid–base status.

2. What is his prognosis?

CASE 21

History

A 59-year-old male with a history of alcohol excess presents to the emergency department with a 3-day history of severe upper abdominal pain. He now also feels very breathless. He admits to drinking up to 100 units of alcohol per week for the past few weeks.

Examination

The patient is in evident distress and appears very unwell. He is tachycardic (120 beats/min) and hypotensive (75/60 mmHg). There is marked epigastric tenderness.

A venous blood test taken on admission reveals a grossly elevated amylase (1890 U/ml) and C-reactive protein (274 mg/L). A chest X-ray on admission is shown in Figure 34.

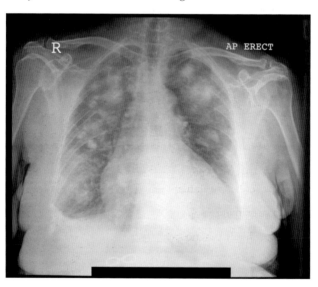

Arterial blood gas		**On 15 L O$_2$ by mask with**
10/08/2005		**reservoir bag**
Unit no.: 45679393		
ID: Daniel Carter		
		Normal
H$^+$	47 nmol/L	(35–45)
pH	7.33	(7.35–7.45)
PCO$_2$	3.24 kPa	(4.7–6.0)
	24.3 mmHg	(35–45)
PO$_2$	10.8 kPa	(> 10.6)
	81 mmHg	(> 80)
Bicarb	14.9 mmol/L	(22–28)
BE	–11.8 mmol/L	(–2–+2)
SPO$_2$	99%	(> 98%)
Lactate	3.1	(0.4–1.5)
K	3.6 mmol/L	(3.5–5)
Na	141 mmol/L	(135–145)
Cl	96 mmol/L	(95–105)
iCa$^+$	0.89 mmol/L	(1–1.25)
Hb	12.0 g/dL	(13.5–18.5)
Glucose	16 mmol/L	(3.5–5.5)

Questions

1. a) Describe his gas exchange.
   b) Describe his acid–base status.

2. What is his approximate FiO$_2$?

3. What is the most likely diagnosis?

CASE 22

History

A 35-year-old woman on a gynaecology ward develops a severe vomiting illness one day after elective sterilisation. She continues to vomit profusely for a further 3 days. Examination of her fluid balance chart reveals that she is failing to keep up with her fluid losses but has not been prescribed intravenous fluids.

Examination

The patient appears dehydrated with reduced skin turgor and dry mucous membranes.

Abdominal examination is unremarkable.

Pulse	100 beats/min
Respiratory rate	10 breaths/min
Blood pressure	160/100 mmHg
Temperature	36.6°C
$O_2\%$	96%

Arterial blood gas		**On air**
23/08/2006		
Unit no.: 27634943		
ID: Jenny Alegranza		
		Normal
H^+	36 nmol/L	(35–45)
pH	7.44	(7.35–7.45)
P_{CO_2}	6.4 kPa	(4.7–6.0)
	48 mmHg	(35–45)
P_{O_2}	11.1 kPa	(> 10.6)
	83 mmHg	(> 80)
Bicarb	32 mmol/L	(22–28)
BE	+4 mmol/L	(–2–+2)
SP_{O_2}	96%	(> 98%)
Lactate	1	(0.4–1.5)
K	3.0 mmol/L	(3.5–5)
Na	133 mmol/L	(135–145)
Cl	91 mmol/L	(95–105)
iCa^+	1.0 mmol/L	(1–1.25)
Hb	11.0 g/dL	(11.5–15.5)
Glucose	5 mmol/L	(3.5–5.5)

Questions

1. a) Describe her gas exchange.
   b) Describe her acid–base status.

2. What electrolyte abnormalities are present?

3. What treatment will correct the acid–base abnormality?

CASE 23

History

An 8-week-old child is brought to the emergency department, with weight loss and projectile vomiting. The parents report that he had an uncomplicated delivery with no postpartum complications. He initially fed well, appeared to be thriving and gave no cause for concern but has deteriorated markedly over the past 2 weeks, vomiting all of his meals and now losing weight.

Examination

The child is agitated, crying and is malnourished. His mucous membranes are dry and on examination of his abdomen a small mass is found in the epigastrium.

Capillary blood gas	**On air**	
05/10/2005		
Unit no.: 28734943		
ID: Richard Barter		
		Normal
H^+	29 nmol/L	(35–45)
pH	7.54	(7.35–7.45)
P_{CO_2}	6.1 kPa	(4.7–6.0)
	45.8 mmHg	(35–45)
P_{O_2}	11.2 kPa	(> 10.6)
	80 mmHg	(> 80)
Bicarb	37.5 mmol/L	(22–28)
BE	+14 mmol/L	(–2–+2)
Sa_{O_2}	99%	(> 98%)
Lactate	1	(0.4–1.5)
K	2.5 mmol/L	(3.5–5)
Na	135 mmol/L	(135–145)
Cl	86 mmol/L	(95–105)
iCa^+	1 mmol/L	(1–1.25)
Hb	18.0 g/dL	(13.5–18.5)

Questions

1. a) Describe his gas exchange.
   b) Describe his acid–base status.

2. Considering the pH and HCO3: is the Pa_{CO_2} higher or lower than you would expect?

3. What is the underlying diagnosis?

CASE 24

History

A 36-year-old pregnant woman on the maternity ward complains of feeling short of breath. She has no other symptoms and no relevant past medical history.

Examination

On examination, the patient is heavily pregnant but appears otherwise well. Examination of her chest reveals no abnormalities.

Pulse	110 beats/min
Respiratory rate	20 breaths/min
Blood pressure	112/100 mmHg
Temperature	36.6°C
O_2%	99%

An ABG is performed.

Arterial blood gas		**On air**
18/08/2005		
Unit no.: 27634943		
ID: Julie Donaldson		
		Normal
H^+	35 nmol/L	(35–45)
pH	7.45	(7.35–7.45)
P_{CO_2}	4.9 kPa	(4.7–6.0)
	35 mmHg	(35–45)
P_{O_2}	4.7 kPa	(> 10.6)
	35 mmHg	(35–45)
Bicarb	24.0 mmol/L	(24–30)
BE	2 mmol/L	(–2–+2)
S_{PO_2}	74%	(> 98%)
Lactate	1	(0.4–1.5)
K	3.6 mmol/L	(3.5–5)
Na	138 mmol/L	(135–145)
Cl	104 mmol/L	(95–105)
iCa^+	1.14 mmol/L	(1–1.25)
Hb	13.0 g/dL	(11.5–15.5)
Glucose	5 mmol/L	(3.5–5.5)

Questions

1. a) Describe her gas exchange.
   b) Describe her acid–base status.

2. What is the most likely explanation for the low PaO_2?

CASE 25

History

A 55-year-old woman on the orthopaedic ward complains of sudden-onset breathlessness and pain on the left-hand side of her chest. She underwent elective knee replacement surgery 4 days previously and has been immobile in bed since the operation. She is otherwise well with no relevant past medical history.

Examination

The patient appears well but slightly short of breath. Other than mild tachycardia and tachypnoea, examination of the cardiovascular and respiratory systems yields no positive findings and there is no clinical evidence of deep-vein thrombosis.

A chest X-ray reveals no abnormalities and an electrocardiogram shows only sinus tachycardia.

Pulse	98 beats/min
Respiratory rate	20 breaths/min
Blood pressure	160/100 mmHg
Temperature	36.6°C
O_2%	99%

Arterial blood gas	**On air**	
10/08/2006		
Unit no.: 27634943		
ID: Jill Archerson		
		Normal
H$^+$	36 nmol/L	(35–45)
pH	7.43	(7.35–7.45)
P_{CO_2}	4.9 kPa	(4.7–6.0)
	37 mmHg	(35–45)
P_{O_2}	12.1 kPa	(> 10.6)
	91 mmHg	(> 80)
Bicarb	25.8 mmol/L	(22–28)
BE	−1.8 mmol/L	(−2–+2)
SP_{O_2}	99%	(> 98%)
Lactate	1	(0.4–1.5)
K	3.8 mmol/L	(3.5–5)
Na	136 mmol/L	(135–145)
Cl	99 mmol/L	(95–105)
iCa$^+$	1.2 mmol/L	(1–1.25)
Hb	10.0 g/dL	(11.5–15.5)
Glucose	5 mmol/L	(3.5–5.5)

Questions

1. a) Describe her gas exchange.
   b) Describe her acid–base status.

2. What is the A–a gradient?

3. Does she require any further investigation?

ANSWERS

1.   a)   Type 1 respiratory impairment (moderate)
       b)   Uncompensated respiratory alkalosis
2.   Yes
3.   Yes

This patient has moderate type 1 respiratory impairment. Hyperventilation is an appropriate response to the hypoxaemia and sensation of dyspnoea and has resulted in a mild alkalaemia (remember that metabolic compensation does not occur in response to *acute* respiratory acid–base disturbance).

The correct management for his condition is supplemental oxygen to correct the hypoxaemia and appropriate antibiotics to treat the infection.

In a patient such as this, with moderate hypoxaemia and no ventilatory impairment, monitoring by pulse oximetry is more appropriate than repeated ABG sampling. Indications for further ABG analysis would include signs of exhaustion or hypercapnia (p. **23**) or a further significant decline in Sao_2.

CASE 2

1. a)   Chronic type 2 respiratory impairment
    b)   Compensated respiratory acidosis
2. Chronic type 2 respiratory impairment due to morbid obesity

At first glance it may be difficult to determine whether this ABG represents respiratory acidosis with metabolic compensation or metabolic alkalosis with respiratory compensation, as both give a high HCO_3 and high Pa_{CO_2}. The best clue is the pH (or H^+) which, although just within the normal range, is on the brink of acidaemia. This would represent overcompensation for an alkalosis and, therefore, suggests an acidosis as the *primary* abnormality (overcompensation does not occur). The mildly impaired oxygenation is consistent with the degree of hypoventilation.

The likeliest cause of chronic type 2 respiratory impairment in this case is severe obesity. Around 20% of individuals with a body mass index greater than 40 have chronic hypercapnia from restricted ventilation (pickwickian syndrome).

CASE 3

1. a) Mild type 1 respiratory impairment (with marked hyperventilation)
   b) Uncompensated respiratory alkalosis
2. Pulmonary embolism

This patient is a young, fit, non-smoker with no history of lung problems but, despite hyperventilating (low Pa_{CO_2}), has a Pa_{O_2} below the normal range, indicating impaired oxygenation. Given the recent long-haul flight and absence of clinical and X-ray abnormalities, the most likely cause of her breathlessness and impaired oxygenation is pulmonary embolism and she must be investigated accordingly.

This is one of the clinical situations where calculation of the A–a gradient can be helpful (more so when the Pa_{O_2} is just within the normal range). As shown below, it is significantly elevated, indicating the presence of V/Q mismatch.

A–a gradient = $PA_{O_2} - Pa_{O_2}$

$PAO2 = (0.21 \times 93.8) - (3.9 \times 1.2)$

$= 19.7 - 4.7$

$= 15$ kPa

A-a gradient = $15 - 10.3$

$= 4.7$ (norm <2.6 kPa)

OR

$PAO2 = (0.21 \times 713) - (29.3 \times 1.2)$

$= 150 - 35$

$= 115$

A-a gradient = $115 - 77$

$= 38$ mmHg (norm <20 mmHg)

CASE 4

1. a) Acute type 2 respiratory failure
   b) Uncompensated respiratory acidosis
2. Opioid toxicity
3. Opioid antagonist

Opioids have a depressant effect upon respiration and may lead to acute ventilatory failure (type 2 respiratory failure). This elderly man has received a large amount of morphine in a short period of time and exhibits pinpoint pupils, making opioid toxicity by far the likeliest cause of his severe ventilatory failure. Since metabolic compensation takes several days to occur, the acute respiratory acidosis has produced a severe acidaemia.

His Pa_{O_2}, though within the normal range, is lower than expected for a patient breathing 28% O_2, and more or less consistent with this degree of hypoventilation.

In addition to basic life support measures, he should be administered an opioid antagonist (e.g. naloxone), to reverse the respiratory depression, then closely monitored to ensure sustained improvement.

CASE 5

1. a) Type 1 respiratory impairment (moderate)
    b) Normal acid-base balance
2. Yes

The above ABG is helpful in guiding the correct treatment for this patient with acute exacerbation of chronic obstructive pulmonary disease. Patients with this condition are often prescribed inadequate oxygen for fear of suppressing hypoxic drive (and thereby depressing ventilation), but this is only an issue in patients with *chronic type 2* respiratory failure (indicated by ↑Pa_{CO_2} and ↑HCO_3). This patient has *type 1* respiratory impairment and will not rely on hypoxic drive.

Although this patient is likely to have a chronically low Pa_{O_2}, the acute deterioration in his symptoms and exercise tolerance suggests a further recent decline from his normal baseline. Importantly, even a small drop in Pa_{O_2} around this level (steep part of O_2–Hb curve) may cause a marked reduction in Sa_{O_2}, compromising O_2 delivery to tissues. Thus O_2 is required both to alleviate symptoms and to prevent the development of tissue hypoxia, and *should not* be withheld for fear of precipitating hypoventilation.

CASE 6

1. a) Acute type 2 respiratory impairment
    b) Uncompensated respiratory acidosis
2. No!

This patient with an acute exacerbation of chronic obstructive pulmonary disease has been struggling to overcome severe obstruction to airflow over a period of hours to days and is now exhausted from the increased work of breathing. As a result, his alveolar ventilation is declining, leading to acute type 2 respiratory failure. This may complicate type 1 respiratory failure from any cause, not just from chronic obstructive pulmonary disease. The rising Pa_{CO_2} is, therefore, *not* due to diminished hypoxic drive and removing his oxygen will *not* correct it. Indeed his FiO_2 should probably be increased (in addition to other treatment) as he remains significantly hypoxaemic.

Remember that, with acute respiratory acidosis, there is no time for metabolic compensation to develop and a dangerous acidaemia develops rapidly. Adequate ventilation must be restored, as a matter of urgency, to correct the Pa_{CO_2}. Possible measures, in this case, include a respiratory stimulant (e.g. doxapram) or, preferably, non-invasive ventilation. If these fail, intubation and mechanical ventilation may be required, if considered appropriate.

CASE 7

1. a)   Type 1 respiratory impairment
    b)   Mild respiratory alkalosis balanced by mild metabolic acidosis
         (likely two primary processes)
2. Aspiration pneumonia
3. Severe

This patient has mild to moderate hypoxaemia despite receiving a high FiO_2 and therefore has severe impairment of oxygenation. The slightly low $Paco_2$ indicates that ventilation is adequate, so this is type 1 respiratory impairment. The probable explanation for the mild metabolic acidosis is lactic acidosis resulting from tissue hypoxia.

The history, examination findings and chest X-ray all suggest a diagnosis of aspiration pneumonia.

This patient is severely unwell and any further decline in her Pao_2 could be catastrophic (on the steep part of the O_2–Hb saturation curve). Her O_2 therapy should be adjusted as necessary to maintain her Sao_2 above 92% and she should be managed on a high-dependency unit with close monitoring for signs of deterioration.

CASE 8

1. a) Chronic type 2 respiratory impairment
   b) Compensated respiratory acidosis
2. PO_2
3. PCO_2 and HCO_3

Acute exacerbation of chronic obstructive pulmonary disease is a common medical emergency and this case illustrates key principles.

1. The $\uparrow Pa_{CO_2}$ shows the patient has type 2 respiratory impairment (ventilatory impairment).
2. The $\uparrow HCO_3$ tells us it is *chronic* type 2 impairment (since metabolic compensation takes time to develop).
3. Even in chronic type 2 impairment, a further *acute* rise in Pa_{CO_2} would lead to an acidaemia. The pH here is normal, so the Pa_{CO_2} has not changed appreciably in the last few days (i.e. there is no acute-on-chronic rise).
4. His Pa_{O_2} *is* likely to have dropped, leading to the increased breathlessness and marked decline in exercise capacity: below a Pa_{O_2} of 8 kPa (60 mmHg) even small falls may cause a major decline in Sa_{O_2} (steep part of the curve).
5. As this patient has chronic hypercapnia, he may rely on hypoxic drive as a stimulus to ventilation.
6. The goal is to ensure adequate oxygenation (we must not ignore his hypoxaemia) without depressing ventilatory drive.

CASE 9

1.   a)   Acute-on-chronic type 2 respiratory impairment
     b)   Partially compensated respiratory acidosis
2.   Excessive supplemental O_2

Care must be taken when prescribing supplemental O_2 to patients with chronic type 2 respiratory failure. The aim is to reverse any recent worsening of hypoxaemia and allow adequate tissue oxygenation, without depressing ventilatory drive through an excessive rise in Pa_{O_2}.

Most authorities recommend controlled O_2 therapy using a fixed-concentration mask at an initial concentration of 24–28%. The response to therapy must be closely monitored with frequent clinical assessment and repeated ABG measurement. Note that pulse oximetry is *not* an adequate substitute for ABG in these circumstances as knowledge of the Sa_{O_2} alone does not permit assessment of ventilatory adequacy.

The latter point is well illustrated in this case as the patient now has life-threatening acute-on-chronic respiratory failure despite a normal Sa_{O_2}. The rising Pa_{CO_2} must be rapidly checked and reversed through improving ventilation. Potential strategies include reducing inspired O_2 concentration, respiratory stimulants or assisted ventilation.

1. a) Mild type 1 respiratory impairment
    b) Normal
2. The Pa_{CO_2} (high end of normal range)
3. Life-threatening attack

This patient has several features of a severe asthma attack but it is the high–normal Pa_{CO_2} that is the most worrying aspect of her presentation and makes it a life-threatening attack. Patients with acute exacerbations of asthma should have a low Pa_{CO_2} on account of the increased respiratory rate and effort (↑alveolar ventilation). A level > 5 kPa (37.5 mmHg) suggests the patient is struggling to overcome the obstruction to airflow and, perhaps, beginning to tire from the effort of breathing. Consequently, her Pa_{CO_2} signals a life-threatening attack.

The intensive care unit should be informed immediately of any patient with acute severe asthma and life-threatening features. Patients must receive intensive treatment and monitoring, including repeated ABG measurements to assess response and identify the need for intubation.

CASE 11

1. a) Hyperventilation (primary)
   b) Uncompensated respiratory alkalosis
2. Low ionized calcium
3. Psychogenic hyperventilation

This is a classic clinical picture of psychogenic hyperventilation. The ABG is entirely in keeping with this diagnosis as it reveals evidence of hyperventilation (low Pa_{CO_2}) with normal oxygenation (normal Pa_{O_2}) and a normal A–a gradient.

Note that the HCO_3 (and BE) is normal as there has been insufficient time for metabolic compensation to occur. Consequently the reduction in Pa_{CO_2} has caused a marked alkalaemia.

Another point to note is that the concentration of ionized calcium in the blood is affected by the pH of the specimen, since H^+ ions compete with calcium for binding sites on albumin and other proteins. Therefore, as the number of H^+ ions drops (alkalaemia), more calcium is bound to albumin, causing serum ionized calcium levels to fall. This is the most likely cause of the numbness and tingling.

Care must be taken in ruling out other cardiovascular and respiratory pathologies before ascribing symptoms of chest pain and shortness of breath to psychogenic hyperventilation.

CASE 12

1. a) Normal – but severe hypoxaemia
   b) Compensated metabolic acidosis
2. Carbon monoxide poisoning
3. Sao_2

Carbon monoxide (CO) poisoning commonly presents with nausea, vomiting, headache and confusion. CO saturations correlate poorly with symptoms but levels above 50% may cause cardiac arrest and seizures.

Why is the patient hypoxaemic?

CO binds to haemoglobin (Hb) with *200 times* the affinity of O_2 so is carried on the Hb molecule (as carboxyhaemoglobin) in preference to O_2. As a consequence, the percentage of Hb saturated with O_2 – the Sao_2 – is markedly reduced in CO poisoning, even when the Pao_2 is very high. Since the overall O_2 content of blood is determined by the Sao_2 and Hb concentration, O_2 delivery to tissues is inadequate (tissue hypoxia), leading to lactic acidosis.

Why does Sao_2 appear to be normal?

Most pulse oximeters are unable to distinguish carboxyhaemoglobin from oxyhaemoglobin, so fail to reflect the true Sao_2 in CO poisoning. In ABG analysis, the Sao_2 is not normally measured but simply *calculated* from the measured Pao_2. The latter parameter is based only on free, unbound O_2 molecules so is unaffected by the presence of CO.

CASE 13

1. a) Hyperventilation – no impairment of oxygenation but hypoxaemia secondary to anaemia (P.18)
    b) Uncompensated respiratory alkalosis
2. Anaemia (Haemoglobin 6.8)
3. Restore haemoglobin (Hb) concentration (e.g. blood transfusion, iron replacement)

This patient appears to have severe anaemia, most likely due to iron deficiency from chronic rectal bleeding. This should be confirmed with a formal laboratory sample ('full blood count').

There is no impairment of ventilation or O_2 transfer so PaO_2 and SaO_2 are normal. However the vast majority of O_2 in blood is carried by Hb, so the overall O_2 *content* of her blood is low.

Hyperventilation is a normal response to the sensation of breathlessness and increases the PaO_2 slightly. However, in the above context, this has very little impact on blood O_2 content as the available Hb molecules are already fully saturated.

For the same reason supplemetal O_2 would also fail to improve O_2 content significantly. Indeed the only effective strategy is to increase Hb concentration. This could be achieved rapidly, by a blood transfusion or more gradually by iron replacement.

CASE 14

1. a) Hyperventilation (secondary)
    b) Partially compensated metabolic acidosis
2. Mesenteric ischaemia

What does the ABG tell us here? There is acidaemia due to a severe metabolic acidosis and the elevated lactate tells us it is a *lactic acidosis*. Lactic acid is produced by tissues receiving an insufficient supply of O_2 but oxygenation is normal (note the Pao_2 is appropriate for an FiO_2 of ~40%) and there are no clinical signs of shock (e.g. hypotension, cold peripheries) suggesting there is no generalised problem of O_2 delivery to tissues.

In fact, the source of lactic acid here is bowel. The patient has mesenteric ischaemia, in which blood supply to the bowel wall is impaired due to occlusion of an artery by a thrombus or embolus. In the absence of an adequate blood supply, bowel tissue becomes hypoxic and must rely on anaerobic metabolism (producing lactate as a byproduct).

Mesenteric ischaemia is a difficult diagnosis to make, as presenting symptoms, signs and routine investigations are all non-specific. The diagnosis should be considered in patients with minimal abdominal examination findings despite severe pain, especially in the presence of a lactic acidosis.

CASE 15

1. a) Hyperventilation (secondary)
    b) Severe metabolic acidosis with partial compensation
2. Anion gap = $(141 + 4.6) - (96 + 6) = 43.6$ (normal = 10–12)
3. Diabetic ketoacidosis

In diabetic ketoacidosis, severe insulin deficiency leads to hyperglycaemia and increased metabolism of fats. The breakdown of fats produces ketone bodies – small organic acids – which provide an alternative source of energy but can accumulate, leading to a profound metabolic acidosis. It is the ketone bodies that account for the raised anion gap.

In this case the acidosis has overwhelmed not only the kidneys' ability to excrete an acid load but also respiratory compensatory mechanisms. There is therefore a severe and dangerous acidaemia despite near-maximal respiratory compensation.

An equally important problem in diabetic ketoacidosis is the profound osmotic diuresis resulting from hyperglycaemia that leads to severe dehydration and electrolyte loss.

CASE 16

1. a) Hyperventilation (secondary)
   b) Severe metabolic acidosis with partial compensation
2. 32
3. Yes

Methanol ingestion can be fatal in doses as small as 30 mL. Methanol is metabolised by the liver to produce formaldehyde and formic acid. Accumulation of formic acid leads to a profound acidosis with a raised anion gap. It also causes ocular toxicity and may result in permanent blindness.

$$\text{Anion gap} = (Na\ \{136\} + K\ \{4.5\}) - (Cl\ \{99\} + HCO_3\ \{9.5\})$$
$$= 140.5 - 108.5$$
$$= 32$$

Treatment for methanol poisoning is complex but often involves the administration of ethanol, which inhibits the conversion of methanol to its more toxic metabolites.

CASE 17

1. a) Slight hyperventilation (secondary)
    b) Compensated metabolic acidosis
2. Anion gap $= (137 + 3.0) - (109 + 18)$
    $$= 138 - 125$$
    $$= 13 \text{ (normal)}$$
3. Renal tubular acidosis (type 1)

The differential diagnosis of normal anion gap acidosis is relatively narrow and, in the absence of diarrhoeal symptoms, renal tubular acidosis (RTA) is the likely cause. The history of renal stones and associated hypokalaemia also supports the diagnosis.

In type 1 RTA, the kidneys fail to to secrete H^+ ions into the urine in exchange for Na^+ ions. This leads to excessive loss of HCO_3 in the urine, resulting in an acidosis. To maintain electroneutrality, extra Cl^- ions are retained (so it is a *hyperchloraemic* acidosis). Because Cl^- is a measured rather than unmeasured anion, there is no increase in the anion gap.

Type 1 RTA is often complicated by renal stones as calcium tends to precipitate in alkaline urine, forming stones.

Hypokalaemia results because Na^+ ions are exchanged for K^+ ions instead of H^+ ions.

CASE 18

1. a) Hyperventilation
   b) Compensated metabolic acidosis *or* metabolic acidosis with concomitant respiratory alkalosis
2. 27
3. Aspirin

Salicylate poisoning may cause both a primary respiratory alkalosis (direct stimulation of the respiratory centre) and a primary metabolic acidosis as salicylate is an acid (it may also promote lactic acid formation). It is therefore not possible to confidently ascertain whether or not the hyperventilation is due to a primary effect of the aspirin or is a response to the metabolic acidosis.

The diagnosis would be confirmed in this instance by taking salicylate levels.

CASE 19

1. a) Hyperventilation (secondary)
   b) Severe metabolic acidosis with partial compensation
2. Hyponatraemia (↓ Na), hyperkalaemia (↑ K), hypoglycaemia (↓ glucose), raised lactate
3. Intravenous corticosteroids

This patient is likely to have adrenal insufficiency, a condition in which the adrenal glands fail to produce sufficient amounts of the hormone cortisol (and, in some cases, aldosterone). It often presents non-specifically with fatigue, malaise, anorexia and weight loss can be easily overlooked or misdiagnosed.

Lack of adrenal hormones causes salt and water depletion and loss of vascular tone which, as in this case, may lead to dramatic circulatory collapse (acute adrenal crisis). The circulatory shock is the cause of the severe lactic acidosis.

Patients also have an inability to mobilise glucose reserves, hence the hypoglycaemia, and characteristic electrolyte abnormalities (↓ Na: ↑ K).

In addition to basic life support and fluid resuscitation, the main intervention likely to improve this patient's condition is the administration of intravenous hydrocortisone.

CASE 20

1. a)   Normal (i.e. satisfactory ventilation and oxygenation being achieved by bag and mask)
    b)   Severe metabolic acidosis (uncompensated)
2. Prognosis   Very poor

In a cardiac arrest case, the ABG has several uses. It allows one to determine the adequacy of ventilation (in this case provided manually by bag and mask), to identify the presence of hyperkalaemia (one of the reversible causes of cardiac arrest) and may provide valuable prognostic information.

Here, despite the evident success of bag and mask ventilation in eliminating CO_2 and oxygenating blood, the patient has a profound lactic acidosis secondary to overwhelming tissue hypoxia. Although this may be multifactorial (e.g. the underlying disease process; hypoxaemia prior to bag and mask ventilation), the most important cause is inadequate tissue perfusion due to loss of cardiac function.

This patient has a grave prognosis. The level of acidosis is unlikely to be compatible with life and, given his unfavourable rhythm (an agonal rhythm does not respond to DC cardioversion and often signifies a 'dying heart'), age and co-morbidities, successful resuscitation is extremely unlikely.

CASE 21

1. a) Type 1 respiratory impairment (severe)
   b) Severe metabolic acidosis with partial compensation
2. 0.6–0.8 (see p. 16)
3. Acute pancreatitis

The diagnosis of acute pancreatitis is based on the history, exam findings and increased serum amylase; the main use of the ABG is in helping to assess illness severity.

The severe lactic acidosis (high anion gap and increased lactate) indicates marked tissue hypoxia. The main cause is impaired blood supply to tissues due to circulatory collapse. This occurs as part of the systemic inflammatory response in pancreatitis and must be urgently corrected with aggressive fluid resuscitation ± vasopressor agents.

A Pa_{O_2} of 10.8 with an Fi_{O_2} of 0.6–0.8 implies severe respiratory impairment, and together with chest X-ray appearances, suggests the development of acute respiratory distress syndrome (an inflammatory lung condition). Although Pa_{O_2} is currently adequate, the patient may require ventilatory support if he deteriorates further or tires from the increased work of breathing.

Finally, the ABG also shows a high glucose and low calcium concentration – both of which are adverse prognostic factors in acute pancreatitis.

The patient should be transferred immediately to a critical care environment for intensive monitoring and supportive treatment.

CASE 22

1. a) Mild type 2 respiratory impairment (compensatory response)
   b) Compensated metabolic alkalosis
2. Electrolytes   Hypokalaemia ($\downarrow$K)
                               Hyponatraemia ($\downarrow$Na)
                               Hypochloraemia ($\downarrow$Cl)
3. Treatment   Fluid and electrolyte replacement

Vomiting causes loss of H^+ ions in gastric juice. The normal response of the kidneys to loss of H^+ ions is increased excretion of HCO_3^- to restore acid–base balance. *So why does this not happen?*

The reason is that persistent vomiting also leads to fluid, Na, Cl and K depletion. In these circumstances the overriding goal of kidneys is salt and water retention.

Under the influence of a hormone called aldosterone, Na^+ ions are retained at the expense of either K^+ or H^+ ions. If K^+ ions were plentiful, H^+ loss could be minimised, but K is also in short supply so both are lost (worsening both the alkalosis and hypokalaemia).

Cl^- depletion also limits HCO_3^- excretion as there must be enough negatively charged ions in blood to balance the positively charged ions (electroneutrality).

Thus, in this case, intravenous replacement of fluid and electrolytes (Na, Cl, K) would allow the kidneys to excrete more HCO_3, correcting the alkalosis.

CASE 23

1. a) Mild type 2 respiratory impairment (compensatory response)
    b) Metabolic alkalosis with partial compensation
2. Lower
3. Pyloric stenosis

Congenital pyloric stenosis is due to hypertrophy of the gastric outflow tract in the first 6 weeks of life. This obstructs flow between stomach and duodenum, leading to projectile vomiting and inability to absorb nutrients.

As in the preceding case, persistent vomiting has caused significant loss of H$^+$ ions, triggering a metabolic alkalosis. Again this is maintained because the associated fluid, Na, Cl and K depletion prevents the kidneys from increasing HCO$_3$ excretion. However, in this case there is a severe alkalaemia for two reasons.

Firstly the metabolic alkalosis is more severe. This is mainly due to the greater duration of vomiting but also because obstruction between stomach and duodenum prevents HCO$_3$ from the duodenum being lost in vomit.

Secondly, there is minimal respiratory compensation. Given the severe alkalaemia, one would predict a greater rise in Pa_{CO_2}. This is probably explained by the child's distress, which provides an additional respiratory stimulus blunting the compensatory response (i.e. a mild primary respiratory alkalosis).

CASE 24

1. a) Appearance of severe type 1 respiratory impairment
    b) Normal acid-base status
2. Explanation   Venous sample

The ABG result suggests severe, life-threatening hypoxaemia but the patient appears clinically well with only mild symptoms and no signs of major respiratory compromise. Moreover, there is a marked discrepancy between the Sa_{O_2} as measured by pulse oximetry (99%) and that calculated on the ABG (74%). By far the likeliest explanation is that the sample was obtained from a vein rather than an artery. A repeat ABG should be performed.

It is important to ensure that an ABG sample is obtained from an artery before using it to assess the Pa_{O_2}. In addition to the points above, non-pulsatile flow and the need to draw back on the syringe at the time of sampling suggest venous blood.

CASE 25

1. a) Normal gas exchange
   b) Normal acid-base status
2. A–a gradient   1.9 kPa/15 mmHg (normal)
3. Yes (must exclude pulmonary embolism)

This case is included to demonstrate the limitation of ABGs and the importance of considering the clinical context. The ABG is entirely normal but the patient is at high risk of pulmonary embolism, given her recent lower-limb orthopaedic surgery and subsequent immobility. Moreover, she has now developed sudden-onset pleuritic pain, breathlessness and tachycardia, unexplained by initial investigations.

While the finding of impaired oxygenation would have lent weight to a diagnosis of pulmonary embolism, a normal ABG result never excludes it. She therefore requires appropriate imaging (e.g. ventilation–perfusion scan or computed tomography pulmonary angiogram) to rule out this diagnosis.

$$\text{A–a gradient} = \quad P_{A}O_2 - P_{a}O_2$$
$$\{(0.21 \times 93.8) - (4.9 \times 1.2)\} - 12.1$$
$$13.9 - 12.1$$
$$= 1.8 \text{ kPa (normal} =< 2.6 \text{ kPa)}$$
or
$$\{(0.21 \times 713) - (37 \times 1.2)\} - 91$$
$$106 - 91$$
$$= 15 \text{ mmHg (normal} < 20 \text{ mmHg)}$$

Index